3.1.78

Good Health Without Drugs

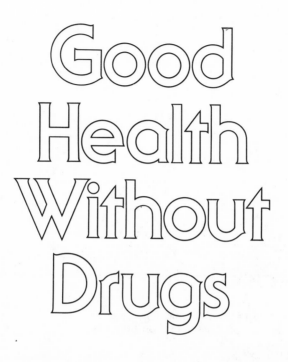

Good Health Without Drugs

Norman D. Ford

St. Martin's Press   New York

Library of Congress Cataloging in Publication Data

Ford, Norman D   1921-
  Good health without drugs.

  Bibliography: p.
  1. Nature, Healing power of. 2. Health.
I. Title.
RZ440.F67   613.2'6   77-9226

ISBN-0-312-33868-6

Contents

2002835

Introduction

This book presents an alternative way to get well and stay well without doctors, drugs, surgery, or hospitals. The philosophy behind it is that we create our own ill health with an unnatural lifestyle that abuses and poisons our bodies. In general, medical science tries to cure disease by treating symptoms with drugs which only tend to intensify the poisons in our bodies that are causing the disease.

Drugs can kill bacteria but they cannot heal. Only the body's own recuperative powers can heal and restore health. Any thinking person might ask: "Why take drugs if they cannot heal and if they increase the toxicity of the body which is sometimes responsible for causing the disease in the first place?"

For the first time in decades, Americans are beginning to ask this very question, particularly in view of the soaring costs of medical care and its frequent lack of success in curing such everyday ailments as arthritis and the common cold.

Centuries before modern medical "advances" were thought of, people were restoring their health through such natural approaches as fasting, exercise and eating natural foods. Today, millions of Americans, disillusioned by the failure of medical science and the huge profits accruing to drug companies and medical equipment manufacturers, are turning to simpler, natural health care systems.

The purpose of this book is to describe Natural Hygiene, probably the most holistic and successful of all natural health care systems. It describes how you can restore your own health and reach a ripe old age free of senility and the whole melancholy catalogue of degenerative diseases that afflict almost everyone who unquestionably accepts our artificial lifestyle.

To be accepted by medical science, a book about Natural Hygiene would require an author with impeccable establishment credentials. Since no qualified scientist or Hygienic practitioner seems willing to produce such a definitive work, the benefits of Natural Hygiene are not widely known. Hundreds of people, given up as "incurable" by the medical profession, are enjoying robust good health today through Natural Hygiene. Thousands more could die while waiting for a book to appear telling them how they also, may be able to restore their health through Natural Hygiene. To prevent any further delay, I have written this book for you, drawing on the entire body of Hygienic knowledge in its preparation.

My own research into the fields of aging and retirement also prompted me to write this book. Wherever I go in the retirement towns of Florida, Arizona, and California, I meet crowds of older Americans—some in wheelchairs, others hobbling around and suffering from a litany of familiar degenerative diseases, almost every last one of which is self-caused. Pick almost any group of one hundred Americans, aged sixty-five and over, and fifty are overweight. Approximately sixty-five suffer from some chronic disease. Fewer than five are in genuine good health.

Sixty-five of every one hundred older Americans are taking medication for their ailments, often three or four different medications. Few, if any, ever tell me that the drugs are improving their condition or making them feel better. Most say the medication merely masks their symptoms.

The colossal realization that, through their own efforts, this immense army of unwell older people could be enjoying radiant good health, and could prolong their lives by many years, motivated me to write this book telling them how.

Of course, Natural Hygiene is not merely for older people. Through living Hygienically, you can achieve optimum health at any age. Many common ailments or diseases can be reversed without surgery or drugs and at minimal expense through Natural Hygiene.

Much of this book is based on studies by eminent authorities in medical science. Almost all of these studies support the validity of Natural Hygiene. Many are openly critical of the medical profession, the food and drug industries, and the government. I have also drawn extensively on the experience of Hygienic practitioners and on the published literature of Natural Hygiene. So many direct or indirect sources have been consulted in researching this book that it is impractical to acknowledge every one.

Natural Hygiene is an extraordinary and exciting program that could change your entire life. For that to happen, of course, you must put into action the principles explained in this book. If you do, you will embark on a revolutionary breakthrough in improving your own personal health. By living Hygienically, you can build vibrant new health and strength and extend your present life expectancy by up to twenty active, healthful years.

But don't take my word for it. This book will tell you what you can expect from Natural Hygiene. You already know what you can expect from living the "good life" and depending on medical care alone. Weigh the pros and cons of both and decide for yourself which health care system offers more.

On frequent occasions in medical history, a thousand learned men with advanced degrees in medicine have been proved wrong by half a dozen laymen who really understood health and how to achieve it. To mention a few: the thalidomide tragedy, the swine flu vaccine fiasco, medically prescribed X-ray treatments that caused cancer, the millions of tonsils that were removed to prevent colds (only to find that removing tonsils caused *more* colds), and the estrogen replacement therapy to ease menopause that turned out to be a high cancer risk.

All these were recommended to the public by thousands of highly qualified men and women holding medical doctorates and other professional credentials. All turned out to be disastrous mistakes that cost hundreds of lives and brought misery to thousands more.

Here, for a change, is a health book by a non-medical writer describing a health care system that uses the body's own recuperative powers to get well. Try it for yourself and see how much better you feel.

Norman D. Ford.
Boulder, Colorado
July 1977

Good Health Without Drugs

1

The Drugless Way to Get Well and Stay Well

Are you plagued by aches, pains and discomforts that get worse despite all the miracle drugs and treatments your doctor prescribes? Are you fed up with medical check-ups that pronounce you fit and well when you look sick and feel tired and run down?

If so, you are probably one of millions of Americans waking up to the fact that drugs, injections, and surgery are not always the medical miracles we have been programmed to believe.

Countless people, after experiencing the hazardous side effects of drugs that often produce little benefit, have felt that there must be a better way. Millions of others, faced with an operation to remove their gallbladder or ulcers, have asked: "Is this the *only* alternative?"

Chiropractic, acupuncture, and homeopathy, among

others, do offer alternative therapies. But they are often no more successful than allopathy (medical treatment). In today's high risk, chemicalized society, a successful non-medical health care system must not only offer a holistic array of natural, biological approaches to better health, but it must also provide an alternative and healthful lifestyle.

A holistic system is one which assumes that body and mind are completely interrelated and that total health is possible only when the entire person is functioning smoothly. Holistic therapy treats the whole person physically, psychologically, emotionally, and spiritually at the same time, using such natural means as nutrition, exercise, fasting, and removing the causes of tension and stress.

Holistic health care concentrates on removing the cause. By contrast, much allopathic practice tends to treat the human organism like an automobile engine, preferring to slap in a new kidney or a plastic aorta instead of seeking out and removing the cause of disease.

But today's overriding health need is an alternative lifestyle that will allow us to survive and reach a ripe old age without getting sick in our stress-filled, poisoned, over-medicated, and under-exercised society.

Such a holistic system has been in existence since 1832. It is called Natural Hygiene, and it is being rediscovered as the only completely effective health-building system that successfully combats not only all the big killer diseases but also most minor ailments from heartburn to low back pains.

Even Hygienists admit that the name, Natural Hygiene, turns people off. But Natural Hygiene has nothing to do with meticulous cleanliness or disinfectants. Hygiene is from the Greek word *hygiēs,* meaning health, and Natural Hygiene simply means the Science of Natural Health.

The purpose of this book is to describe the Natural Hygiene system and to explain how you can use it to improve and maintain your own health.

Natural Hygiene offers a simple way to:

●Eliminate almost all risk of getting cancer by approximately 50 percent and continue reducing this risk as you become older.

●Increase your mental abilities and become more alert.

●Bring your weight to its ideal level and keep it there without dieting for the rest of your life.

●Enjoy robust good health for the remainder of your life with a minimum of colds, flu, and other common ailments. Some allergies may also disappear.

●Banish almost all common digestive complaints such as constipation and irregularity, acid indigestion, belching, heartburn, bloating, gas, bad breath, and body odors.

●Conquer chronic fatigue and weariness and regain the energy and stamina of your youth.

●Boost sexual vigor and become more attractive to the opposite sex.

●Improve your eyesight and very possibly your taste, smell, and hearing also.

●Give yourself a slim, well-built body and a more youthful appearance.

●Replace stress, fear, and anxiety with a permanent feeling of relaxed calm and tranquillity.

●Make your skin clearer and your hair full of luster—both signs of inner good health.

●End most types of headaches as well as most other aches and pains, including most forms of backache and low back pain.

•Cut out almost all doctor, drug, and hospital bills and substantially reduce dental expenses.
•Give yourself an entirely new, health-filled lifestyle full of exciting new adventures and opportunities.

A miracle? Not to a Hygienist. For Natural Hygiene recognizes that all of the ailments listed above are due to a single cause. The principle of Natural Hygiene is to remove this cause, allowing the body's own natural recuperative powers to heal the organism and return it to health. Excluding inherited and congenital defects and injuries, *the cause of almost all human ailments is toxemia.*

Toxemia results from toxins entering and poisoning the human organism and depleting its energy. Toxemia is the result of abuse of the body by direct intake of drugs or stimulants; eating unhealthy food high in fats, cholesterol, and refined carbohydrates; overeating; getting insufficient sleep and rest; lack of exercise, sunshine, and fresh air; emotional stress, tension, insecurity, and polluted food, air, and water.

Gradually, toxemia weakens the body until the immunological system breaks down and an infectious disease or cancer gains a hold, or until the arteries become clogged with fats and cholesterol, paving the way for one or more of a variety of degenerative diseases such as hypertension, heart attack, and stroke. Toxins such as asbestos or chlordane are just two among thousands of products of our technological society that can enter the body and, over a period of years, induce cancer. Cigarette smoke and alcohol are direct causes of toxemia as are coffee, tea, chocolate, salt, aspirin, all prescription and non-prescription drugs, and radiation from X-rays,

TV sets, microwave ovens, and fluorescent lights.

Cancer and heart disease do not strike at random. They usually occur in people debilitated by years of toxemia, their energy sapped by years of unhealthy living. Wherever disease occurs, Hygienists consider it a symptom of an underlying condition of toxemia. Once toxemia exists, a disease will tend to break out in whichever part of the organism happens to be weakest. If the immune system is weakened, the body's white cells may be unable to fight off infectious diseases such as influenza or pneumonia. If the respiratory organs are weak, one may get bronchitis or asthma. If the digestive system is weak, it may be gallstones, colitis, or ulcers.

Since most diseases are symptoms of toxemia, Hygienists are not overly concerned with diagnosis. Hygienists belive in only one basic disease, one cause, and one road back to health. The disease is toxemia, the cause is abuse of the body, and the remedy is to restore the body's biological necessities so that its natural recuperative powers can go to work and restore health to the whole person—it's as simple as that.

Staying healthy *is* incredibly simple and easy. Through Natural Hygiene, you can attain a level of fitness, mental alertness and emotional well-being beyond your wildest expectations. Few adult Amercians have ever experienced real health. If you are under seventy and not active, completely free of disease, and filled with glowing good health and vibrant energy, you may be average but you are far below normal. The average physician today will pronounce you fit and well if you register normal in routine diagnostic tests and show no signs of disease. But lack of disease symptoms is a negative form of good health. Thousands of men have been given a clean bill of health by their doctors only to collapse a week later with a heart attack.

The kind of health Hygienists talk about means feeling great and well all of the time: having no bad days or depressing experiences: having almost boundless energy and stamina: and functioning actively to a ripe old age without sickness or senility.

That this isn't the kind of health doctors mean is shown by the results of an automated battery of tests given to 2,500 physicians over a period of several years at A.M.A. conventions. Made on physicians aged thirty to sixty-five, the tests revealed that 20 percent showed symptoms of diabetes, 30 percent had above-average cholesterol levels, 12 percent showed possible indications of gout, and another 15 percent showed possible indications of heart trouble. While thousands of doctors *have* given up smoking and foods high in fat and cholesterol, the personal health standards of the average physician fall far short of those of the average Hygienist.

In many ways, the philosophy of Natural Hygiene is diametrically opposed to that of medicine. Hygiene offers no cures. By contrast, allopathy attempts to cure diseases which Hygienists consider mere symptoms of a deeper underlying condition. Thus Hygienists accuse doctors of Band-Aid medicine, of treating symptoms with palliatives instead of finding and removing the cause of disease.

In place of cures, Hygiene offers only a way to improve and recover one's health. Obviously, health and disease cannot exist simultaneously. In many cases, as a person's health improves, aches, pains, and ailments may gradually slip away and disappear. Hygienists are quick to point out that Natural Hygiene is not one of the healing arts.

What, then, is Natural Hygiene?

It is a health care system that recognizes man's complete dependence on Nature and it aids Nature in restoring health.

It holds that the human organism is self-healing if in a toxic-free state and supplied with its natural requirements, such as fresh air, pure water, sunshine, exercise, wholesome food, rest, relaxation, emotional calm, and security.

It teaches how to detoxify the system by fasting so that it can become self-sufficient in restoring health.

It teaches how to live correctly with our biological heritage so that the organism remains free of toxins and, as a result, free of most of the diseases and ailments which plague mankind.

Natural Hygiene advocates a vegetarian diet of fresh, living foods such as fruits, vegetables, nuts, and seeds. While not entirely holistic—it lacks any spiritual approach—most Hygienists develop a close relationship with Nature that borders on the spiritual.

The Advantages of Assuming Responsibility for Your Own Health

Since diagnosis is relatively unimportant, and since drugs only intensify toxemia, and removal of organs is un-holistic, physicians receive little business from Hygienists. Only in the unlikely event of a Hygienist suspecting cancer or, perhaps, problems of sight, might he normally consult a physician. But Hygienists rarely suffer from such ailments. Instead, Hygienists take full responsibility for their own state of health. Should a Hygienist need advice, he would consult a Hygienic practitioner.

Most Americans, by contrast, have a passive attitude

7

towards health and medicine. Here I am, they tell their physican. Drug me, cut me open, make me well. They are actually disappointed if the doctor does not write a prescription or suggest treatment or an operation.

To many Americans, health protection means taking out medical insurance so that they can die in an intensive care unit stuck full of sensors and other Frankenstein-like paraphernalia, that they can prolong their lives a few miserable years on a kidney dialysis machine, or perhaps have their cancerous lower organs removed so that bowel and bladder movements eject into a plastic bag through an opening in the side.

The idea that most diseases are self-caused and that they can be prevented, or possibly reversed, by taking responsibility for one's own health, is a concept totally alien to most Americans. Somehow we've been brainwashed into believing that we are incapable of making intelligent decisions or of assuming responsibility for our own health.

You should not exercise, fast, or change your diet without first obtaining your doctor's permission, we are constantly told. Admittedly, a diabetic or anyone under medical care or with permanent damage to the heart or vascular or other system should certainly have medical approval first. But this philosophy discourages the rest of us from taking an active role in caring for our health. By making us believe we are merely passive observers of our own health, unable to play an active role in getting better, medical science has established a monopoly on health care and its profits.

By contrast, Natural Hygiene makes you personally responsible for your own health. Hygienists assert the right to make all decisions regarding their own health and to take an active role in restoring it.

What Proof Is There That Natural Hygiene Really Works?

Although some M.D.s have recognized the merits of Natural Hygiene and practice it, few if any medically acceptable studies have been made to substantiate its claims.

Although there are several million vegetarians in America today, possibly only 50,000 people practice some degree of Natural Hygiene. About 2,500 belong to the American Natural Hygiene Society (ANHS), a Chicago-based organization with a nationwide membership and regional chapters. The ANHS publishes its own literature and books which give complete instructions on diet, exercise, and other aspects of the system.

Basic Hygienic practices include a raw food vegetarian diet consisting of fresh fruits, vegetables, nuts, and seeds; optional short or long fasts for detoxification and breaking habits such as smoking and drinking; and a daily exercise program geared to individual ability.

After attending two national conventions and meeting several hundred ANHS members, our opinion is that at least 10 percent of the ANHS membership fail to exercise daily or to strictly observe the diet and other aspects. Yet we found that most of those who do adhere to Hygienic principles are walking advertisements for the system. . .suntanned, slim, youthful, and filled with vibrant good health and boundless energy until well into their eighties and even nineties.

In addition, an estimated 47,500 non-ANHS members

practice some degree of Natural Hygiene. Among these are followers of author John Tobe, whose many books recommend a lifestyle that differs from Natural Hygiene only in that fasting is not employed and that whole grain cereals are also a part of the diet. Many Hygienists, including some ANHS members, also supplement their diet with cooked whole grain cereals while other Hygienists cook some of their starchier vegetables such as potatoes and turnips. But the ANHS does not approve of cereals or cooked foods.

Rounding out the picture are a dozen or so Hygienic health resorts and fasting institutions dotted around the country and in Mexico. Also, in Florida there is a sizeable commune of retired Hygienists who are largely self-sufficient. Hygienists, by and large, are a scattered, rather loose-knit group, difficult to identify, appraise, and keep track of.

By contrast, medically supervised studies have been made of three other very closely related groups, with clear and unmistakable results. These groups are: 1. the long-lived peoples of Abkhasia in the U.S.S.R. and of Vilcabamba in Ecuador; 2. the California Seventh Day Adventists; and 3. participants in the health rehabilitation programs of the Longevity Research Institute in Santa Barbara, California.

The World's Longest Lived People Follow a Hygienic Lifestyle

The Abkhasians are a society of hill farmers living in an isolated region of the Caucasus Mountains. In this peaceful Black Sea region, people live the kind of life that most Hygienists dream about. The Abkhasians work hard outdoors all day, raising and eating their own organically grown fruits, vegetables, and cereals. They are far from the tensions and pressures of modern society and in an environment still completely unpolluted.

In almost every sense, the Abkhasians are practicing Natural Hygiene. Their entire lifestyle is actually a holistic health care system guaranteed to make them thrive. Prior to about 1930, the Abkhasians were less affluent than they have become since the Russian Revolution. In earlier years, they were almost completely vegetarian. Nowadays, about 30 percent of their diet consists of low-fat dairy foods such as yogurt in addition to some mutton, chicken or goat—all raised under natural conditions and free of the high fat content and pesticide residues so common in America.

All of their food is consumed fresh, with meat either broiled or roasted. They eat a variety of cereals and an abundance of fresh fruits and vegetables. Honey is used in place of sugar, a parched corn cereal in place of bread.

As might be expected, the Abkhasians enjoy almost perfect health throughout their long, active lives. They are among the world's longest-lived peoples. One Abkhasian who worked in the fields until he was 163 years old, died recently aged 168. Abkhasian youngsters grow up expecting to live at least one hundred healthful years and most Abkhasians consider themselves still youthful until well into their eighties. The proportion of centenarians in Abkhasia is almost seven times greater than in America.

Abkhasians remain physically active throughout their lives and they never retire or cease to work. Many Abkhasians aged ninety and over have blood pressure readings below 110/75. And at age ninety or over, their cholesterol level averages only 92 mg. per cent—compared with 240 mg. per cent for the average American aged fifty-five.

Numerous investigations and studies have been made to confirm the extreme age attained by Abkhasians and to find out how they stay so fit and well. Of Abkhasians aged ninety and over, 40 percent of men and 30 percent of women have almost perfect eyesight. In one study of 123 Abkhasians aged one hundred and over, there were no reported cases of illness or cancer during nine years of observation.

Soviet cardiologist Dr. David Kakiashuili and others have probed into every detail of Abkhasian diet and habits. They found, for instance, that Abkhasian males over eighty consume 1,800 calories per day, of which only 50 grams is fat. The typical American, by contrast, consumes 3,300 calories of which 157 grams is fat. Dr. Kakiashuili also found that the longevous people do have heart attacks but they are almost invariably "silent" and unnoticed. Due to the low fat level of their diet and their continuous physical activity, they are able to develop collateral blood supplies to the heart which prevent muscle atrophy should a coronary artery become clogged.

The Vilcabambans were, until very recently, a smaller group of equally healthy and long-lived hill farmers living in a remote Andean valley. Church baptism and death records show that, on a per capita basis, their rate of centenarians until recently was higher than Abkhasia's.

What has placed all this in the past tense is a new highway that was put through to Vilcabamba in late 1974. Until then, Vilcabambans were almost completely vegetarian. But the new highway has brought sugar, white rice, white flour, and trichinosis-filled pork. And in just two short years, the death rate in Vilcabamba has soared by 30 percent.

New roads to neighboring villages that also had a high proportion of longliving people have also destroyed the old stress-free lifestyle. But the road has not yet reached Surunuma. In 1976, this tiny village had thirty-eight people aged eighty or over, including several centenarians. Instead of eating the devitalized foods that have killed almost all the centenarians in Vilcabamba, the Surunumans still live on their traditional vegetarian foods. Amazingly, the daily food intake of these active oldsters is only 1,200 calories, of which only 1-2 percent is fat.

A third group of super-healthy, long-lived hill farmers reside in Hunza, a remote Himalayan valley in Pakistan. The Hunzas, too, have been vegetarian. But inroads of civilization have brought sugar and other depleted foods to Hunza and the traditional lifestyle is rapidly disappearing.

Yet Alexander Leaf, M.D., a professor at Harvard Medical School, who in the early 1970s visited all three regions when they were still unchanged, was more impressed by the extreme fitness of the longevous people than by their extreme ages. In all three areas, he found that people aged ninety and over were robust and active, nimble and extremely energetic.

Commented Dr. Leaf: "The weight of current medical opinion would concur that a diet such as that described for Hunza and Vilcabamba would delay development of atherosclerosis—that is, fatty deterioration of the arteries of the heart."

Atherosclerosis, or hardening of the arteries, is the basic condition which leads to high blood pressure, stroke, heart attack, kidney disease, and a host of other ills that plague Americans. It is the most common form of toxemia found in western, meat-eating nations.

It is worth noting that most long-lived Abkhasians were almost completely vegetarian until age sixty or over. For all practical purposes, all three longevous peoples lived all or most of their lives on a vegetarian diet.

It is true that in these societies, a few people do smoke and many enjoy a drink or two during celebrations. But considering all aspects of their lives—diet, rugged exercise, freedom from tension and deadlines—their lifestyles more closely approach the ideals of Natural Hygiene than the actual daily routines of many American Hygienists.

California's Amazingly Healthful Seventh Day Adventists and Utah's Mormons

Though it does not necessarily recommend fasting or raw food, the Seventh Day Adventist Church (SDA) does endorse vegetarianism and a healthful lifestyle for its members that in many respects is almost identical with Natural Hygiene.

A study of 35,460 Adventists living in California, undertaken in a joint government-Adventist investigation, found that Adventists live, on average, seven years longer than the general population. Compared to the general California population, 70 percent fewer Adventists die from cancer, 68 percent fewer from respiratory diseases, 88 percent fewer from T.B., 85 percent fewer from emphysema, 46 percent fewer from stroke, 60 percent fewer from heart disease, 93 percent fewer from cirrhosis of the liver, and 35 percent fewer from accidents.

The SDA population abstains from smoking and drinking and most Adventists avoid the use of stimulatns, condiments, and spices. But only half are estimated to be strict vegetarians and of these many are lacto-ovo vegetarians, meaning that they also eat dairy products and eggs. Nonetheless, almost all Adventists abstain from alcohol and pork, and their overall use of meat and coffee is well below average.

Other studies reveal that Adventists have fewer dental problems and that Adventist women have significantly lower post-menopausal rates of cancer of the breast, ovary, and uterus. Probably due to abstinence from coffee, the SDA rate of bladder cancer is also well below average.

The recommended Adventist diet consists largely of vegetables, fruits, whole grain cereals and nuts, and SDAs tend to avoid refined foods. As a result, the overall Adventist consumption of fats, cholesterol, animal proteins and refined carbohydrates—such as sugar, and white bread—is far below the American norm. One investigation showed that the SDA diet contains 50 percent more fiber and 25 percent less fat than the U.S. average and fewer food additives and preservatives.

While much of the Adventists' startling reduction of cancer and heart disease may be attributed to their ban on smoking and their reduced intake of fat, other investigations show that a vegetarian diet may be responsible for much of their success. Probing further into SDA health records, Dr. Roland Phillips, of Loma Linda University, found that Adventists who did get heart disease or bowel cancer ate more fish, meat, and dairy products than the average SDA. Adventists who suffered cancer of

15

the breast or bowel were also found to have eaten more fried and refined foods than the average SDA. Adventists who did *not* get cancer were reported to have eaten more green, leafy vegetables and plant protein.

The population of Utah is 72 percent Mormon and health records for Utah show an overall cancer death rate 22 percent below the national average. While Mormons do eat meat in moderation, the Mormon *Words of Wisdom* forbids use of all stimulants, tobacco, and addictive drugs and extols eating fruits, vegetables, and grains. This lifestyle reduces the Mormons' risk of cancer by 50 percent.

Instead of living in remote villages in the Andes or Caucasus, these groups are living right here among us in America. One explanation is that their diet, religion and way of life provide both Adventists and Mormons with what amounts to a holistic system of natural health care comparable to Natural Hygiene.

Killer Diseases Reversed by Fat-Free Diet

In 1976, for the first time in medical history, hardening of the arteries—the leading cause of heart disease and stroke—was reversed in humans without drugs or surgery. This remarkable feat was achieved by nutritionist Nathan Pritikin, Director of the Longevity Research Institute at Santa Barbara, California.

We say remarkable, but although this was the first time that atherosclerosis reversal was medically supervised and documented, Hygienists have been doing the same thing for decades.

This is not to slight Pritikin's achievement. Taking a group of sixteen people, six of whom were candidates for by-pass surgery and one for claudication, Pritikin's methods so improved their condition that after his thirty-day session, none of the seven needed surgery.

At the end of the thirty-day live-in session, out of seven original cases of angina, only two remained; of five cases of high blood pressure, none remained; the one case of emphysema was so improved that no further medication was required; two cases of diverticulosis required no further medication; of three cases of arthritis, only one remained; the single diabetic was able to reduce his insulin from thirty-five to eighteen units daily; one case of chronic constipation disappeared; one case of claudication, controlled by drugs for twenty years, was able to increase treadmill performance by 788 percent; four cases of partial kidney failure recovered away; and of five cases of undiagnosed diabetes, only one remained. Out of thirty-eight different medications taken by the group, only five were necessary at the end of the session and of these, the daily dosage was reduced by 25-50 percent.

Each of the sixteen participants lost weight, reduced cholesterol levels by 20-35 percent, and triglycerides blood fat levels by an average 31.86 percent. Blood pressures also dropped significantly.

During a following thirty-day session, twelve drug-controlled hypertensives (people with high blood pressure) started with an average blood pressure of 141/82. After thirty days, none of the group was on drugs and the average blood pressure had dropped to 119/67—a 100 percent reversal of hypertension entirely by natural methods.

Pritikin's system is based entirely on diet and exercise. In the average U.S. diet, 40-45 percent of the calories are derived from fats. Even diets advised by heart specialists are 35 percent fat. But only 10 percent of Pritikin's diet is fat, with the balance consisting of 10 percent protein and 80 percent complex carbohydrates, meaning vegetables, fruits, and whole grain cereals. No supplements, vitamins, or minerals are added, and there is no coffee, tea, sugar, salt, caffeine, or nicotine.

This diet compares very closely with those of the Abkhasians, Vilcabambans, and Hygienists. The aim is to reduce the cholesterol level in the bloodstream and thereby to eliminate atherosclerosis. Pritikin considers that any cholesterol level above 160 produces artery damage. The average U.S. physician considers anything under 194 as permissible, and even readings of 220 are not considered exceptionally high. Instead of three meals a day, participants are served eight to nine smaller meals to reduce the stress of digestion and the sudden increase in blood sugar resulting from large meals.

For exercise, Pritikin's groups walk or jog five to fifteen miles or more daily, depending on the individual. As participants progress, they are allotted hillier routes to force a continuous challenge.

An essential feature of the program is a series of twenty-two ninety-minute evening lectures during which participants learn how to eat and exercise for the rest of their lives. The lifetime maintenance diet allows up to one pound of animal protein each week. Pritikin finds that when someone exceeds this amount, cholesterol deposits invariably occur in the arteries.

Though Pritikin's program was originally tailored to reverse advanced cardiac cases, it has also been able to reverse cases of diabetes, gout, senility, and arthritis. In fact, his results closely approximate those reported by practitioners at Hygienic institutions. And though not entirely holistic, his system so closely parallels the exercise and dietary principles of Natural Hygiene that differences seem virtually negligible.

Hygienists Are Safe From Most Killer Diseases

If the results of these three Hygienic type lifestyles sound impressive, remember that Natural Hygiene goes further than all of them put together. First, Hygiene employs fasting that eliminates toxemia by purifying the bloodstream and tissues. If necessary, fasting is also employed to shed weight and is also highly effective in reversing addiction to tobacco, alcohol, and other drugs. Secondly, the Hygienic diet is not only completely vegetarian—no dairy foods or eggs—but is composed only of fresh, living foods.

As Dr. Roland Phillips' studies showed, the more purely vegetarian their diet, the lower were the health risks of the Adventists. The Hunzas and Vilcabambans were almost completely vegetarian, while almost all Abkhasian centenarians have been vegetarians for most of their lives. Too, the Longevity Research Institute diet is largely vegetarian.

Heart disease, cancer, diabetes, arthritis, and other common diseases that are almost epidemic in America have been virtually unknown in less affluent, vegetarian societies such as Hunza or Vilcabamba.

Hygienists believe that foods should be eaten fresh and whole, exactly as they come from the ground or off the tree. Drying is the only type of processing acceptable. Foods that have been canned, frozen, or otherwise embalmed are nutritionally weakened. Only by eating foods in their raw, uncooked, and unfragmented state are all enzymes, vitamins, minerals, proteins, fats, carbohydrates, and other essential components preserved intact.

Cooking deaminizes some proteins, converts starches

19

to simple sugars, and changes oils and fats to toxic and often carcinogenic substances. These facts are borne out by the work of Dr. Leo Wattenburg at the University of Minnesota Medical School who, through experiments on rats, demonstrated that eating fresh vegetables, citrus, beans, or seeds causes production of enzymes that help protect the body against cancer.

Evidence is also emerging which shows that fresh, uncooked foods, even meat and dairy foods, deposit appreciably less cholesterol in the arteries than cooked foods. Experiments on cats carried out in the 1940s by the late Dr. Francis M. Pottinger Jr., also demonstrates the negative effects of feeding animals on cooked foods. Cats fed on raw meat and milk thrived while those fed cooked meat and heated milk became lethargic and unwell.

When digested, uncooked foods are predominantly alkaline, a condition considered essential to health. Cooked foods, including beans and cereals, are acid-forming (accounting for the tremendous consumption of antacid tablets). For this reason, most Hygienists eat grains and beans only when sprouted.

Eating the Hygienic way typically means starting the day with a large, delicious fruit salad. Lunch might be a vegetable salad with potatoes, carrots, and other starchy vegetables. Dinner would probably consist of a large vegetable salad with avocado, mixed nuts, and sunflower seeds. For a snack, you could eat two or three oranges.

Far from being confined to a dull diet, a Hygienist can choose his foods from almost the entire range of the vegetable kingdom. Compared to just a few types of meats, fish, poultry, and dairy foods, you'll find literally dozens of fruits, vegetables, nuts, and seeds to choose from.

One thing is abundantly clear. High in fiber, low in fats, and with a zero level of cholesterol, the Hygienic diet rates tops in supplying every nutritional need, including a very adequate amount of complete protein. Far from criticizing vegetarianism, eminent nutritionists are beginning to realize that the human organism was not designed to digest animal fats and proteins, or highly refined supermarket foods.

In the May 1976 issue of *Today's Health,* author Nicholas Gonzalez wrote: "Evidence indicates that the typical American diet, loaded with fat, sugar, and highly refined foods, is responsible for our high rates of intestinal and breast cancer. How can a person's diet have such serious consequences? The fact is that our bodies just aren't adapted to the kind of food we eat."

Gonzalez points out that for a million years our ancestors lived on a diet of fruits, berries, herbs, roots, and wild animal meat, which is much leaner than feed-lot beef and contains far fewer saturated fats. Agriculture is only 8,000 years old, he says, which is hardly much time in the scale of evolution. Our diet has changed too much and too quickly for our bodies to adapt.

Dr. Ernst Wynder, President of the American Health Foundation, also believes the fat content of our diet is responsible for our high colon cancer rate. Says Dr. Wynder: "It is obvious from the work in arteriosclerosis[1] that our human body was not engineered to handle the kind of food we give it today, particularly since we are a sedentary population."

Yet the twelve-ounce steak continues to be routine for millions of Americans on Saturday night.

---

[1]Arteriosclerosis is a generic term for hardening of the arteries; atherosclerosis means hardening of the arteries due to fatty deposits such as cholesterol.

2

Why Hygienists Don't Get Sick
The Causes of Toxemia and How
to Avoid Them

Carmela B. was fifty-seven when she was diagnosed as diabetic. She was examined and treated by three different physicians and told she must take insulin for the rest of her life.

After one year on insulin, Carmela had all the usual symptoms of a diabetic. Her mouth was dry and she experienced continual thirst. She was forced to urinate at frequent intervals. She was often constipated. The skin on her mid-section became rough and dry. And her ankles were swollen with edema.

A year after Carmela became diabetic, a friend recommended that she spend a vacation at Villa Vegetariana, a Hygienic Health School and fasting institution at Cuernavaca, Mexico. Shortly after her arrival, the resident physician placed Carmela on a fast. For ten days she took nothing but pure mountain water. On the tenth day, she broke the fast.

Carmela felt like a completely new person. After a few days on a diet of vegetables, fruits, nuts, and seeds, her thirst was gone and her mouth remained comfortably moist. She began to urinate normally. Her bowel movements became easy and regular. The skin on her midsection turned soft and smooth. And her edema disappeared.

According to her testing kit, Carmela was no longer diabetic. Subsequent tests confirmed a complete reversal of her diabetes. Since her fast, she has taken no insulin nor medication of any kind. She has faithfully followed the Hygienic lifestyle and is now leading a completely normal life.

Like all degenerative diseases, diabetes mellitus caused by toxemia, in this case a high level of fat in the blood—the result of a diet high in fats, cholesterol, animal protein, and refined carbohydrates. By simply cutting off the intake of fats, and allowing the body to eliminate its surplus fat, Carmela's blood fat level returned to normal and her diabetes promptly vanished. Her case is not unique.

Too much fat is one of the causes of a toxemic condition in the body that inhibits the production of the hormone insulin. This prevents the body's cells from burning sugar for energy. Instead, the cells obtain their energy from fat and protein. In doing so, the cells give off toxic by-products which intensifies the condition of toxemia to the point where coma and death sometimes occur.

The toxins which cause toxemia are extraneous poisons and metabolic wastes which enervate the body's reserves of energy and cause a variety of degenerative and other diseases and ailments. Besides toxic substances which enter the body through the digestive system or lungs, a surfeit of the body's own by-products can be equally lethal.

When cholesterol is deposited in the arteries, it is a form of toxemia that can lead to a heart attack. But cholesterol is also synthesized by the body for its own use. However, research has shown that the beta type cholesterol, which causes atherosclerosis, heart attacks and strokes, is deposited in the arteries only when transported by protein compounds that are low in denity. Low density lipoproteins (LDLs) are another form of toxemia that results from lack of exercise and a diet high in animal fats.

A person with a high cholesterol level coupled with a high rate of LDLs is in an advanced stage of toxemia with a correspondingly high risk of a heart attack. By contrast, in a person who exercises regularly and who eats a low fat diet, cholesterol is transported by high density protein compounds. High density lipoproteins are non-toxic and actually work to clear cholesterol out of the arteries and into the liver where it is degraded and expelled.

Biological functions aside, heart attacks and strokes are the direct result of toxemia caused by lack of exercise and a diet high in animal fats. For simplicity's sake, through the remainder of this book, we shall refer to a person in this condition as suffering from a high level of cholesterol.

Another of the most widespread forms of toxemia in Americans is a high triglycerides level, a high level of lipids (fats) in the bloodstream. It is caused by eating vegetable oils as well as animal fats.

A person with both high cholesterol and high triglycerides levels has a heart attack risk five times greater than with a high cholesterol level alone. The excessively toxic condition caused by both a high cholesterol and a high triglycerides level is further intensified when another toxin, such as cigarette smoke, is added. The overall risk is multiplied further when a person fails to exercise.

Another very common toxemic condition in American are carcinogenic (cancer causing) residues in our organs and tissues. Over a period of years, and in cooperation with stress and poor nutrition, carcinogens may eventually cause mutations in the genes of body cells and make them cancerous.

The frantic pace of daily living in our complex society creates constant stress-filled situations. The body reacts to stress with such undesirable emotions as hatred, anger, fear, anxiety, and envy. These emotions trigger the glands to release a flood of hormones that, in primitive times, tensed the body to either fight off the offending cause of stress or to run away from it. Since nowadays we can do neither, we are left filled with tension.

Tension is a form of toxemia that makes us feel uptight and causes headaches. But far worse, it upsets our immunological balance. When this happens, the system's predatory white cells become too lethargic to seek out and destroy invading virus and bacteria. The result is lowered resistance to coughs, colds, flu, and pneumonia, and very possibly a heightened risk of cancer.

Toxemia also depletes our physical energy and our animal enjoyment of active exercise. Without abundant exercise, our hearts become flabby and our arteries and muscles weaken. Leading exercise physiologists have found that the classic symptoms of old age are not due to aging at all but to lack of physical activity. They also report that up to 85 percent of all back troubles are merely due to sedentary living encouraged by toxemia.

Our Health-Wrecking Lifestyle

The direct cause of toxemia is our lifestyle. To believe in America's "Good Life" is to buy a one-way ticket to self-destruction. Most of the goals Madison Avenue holds up as desirable are highly hazardous to health. Beef, Scotch, coffee, cigarettes, ice cream, luxury cars, soft living, and the desire to buy more and more things overload our circuits with toxins and tensions. The American system is stacked 100 percent against good health and long life.

One in every twelve Americans has some form of digestive disease, and one of every three major operations is for ulcers, gallstones, colitis, or other digestive ailments. The average American male has one chance in five of having a heart attack before sixty. One in every four Americans is stricken with cancer, and almost one in five dies of it. Approximately one American in four has some form of arthritis. Latest estimates show that one in every six American adults may have hypertension, and approximately the same proportion show some degree of diabetic symptoms. Weak kidneys are commonplace. By age fifty-five, one American in two has lost all his teeth and is suffering from a chronic disease.

Our national ill-health statistics are trying to tell us something about our lifestyle and diet. What they are saying is that you have to be smart and determined to survive.

Can We Live Safely In Our Carcinogenic Society?

Dr. Irving Selikoff, head of the Environmental Health Department at New York's Mount Sinai Hospital, and his associates, found that 80-85 percent of all cancer is caused by man-made products and chemicals needed to support the industrial lifestyle. The earth's air, water, and soil are filled with traces of cancer-causing plastics, asbestos, aerosol spray chemicals, smoke, talcum powder, and dozens of other pollutants. Cancers we are seeing now stem from cancer-producing agents introduced into the environment twenty or thirty or even forty years ago. Right now we are determining the health of our children in the year 2,000. The list of carcinogens is growing daily.

Considerable evidence exists that much of the food being served in school lunch programs will give children cancer of the colon in twenty to thirty years. The U.S. already has one of the world's largest rates for colon cancer. So chemicalized is our environment that every time we breathe, eat, drink, or touch something, we may be risking our lives.

However, almost all the hazards are limited to the "Good Life" and its way of living and eating. If we are smart and determined, we *can* survive. Through Natural Hygiene, we can build up and safeguard our health instead of letting the "Good Life" tear it down.

The first lesson in Natural Hygiene is to learn to recognize the high risk factors in our society so that we can avoid them.

Farmers Are Waging Chemical Warfare on The U.S. Population

In the early 1970s, the Food and Drug Administration (FDA) banned the use of cholorinated pesticides and replaced them with organo-phosphorous compounds. But residues of DDT and the more recently banned polychlorinated biphenyls (PCBs) are in the tissues of almost every American, and they are likely to remain in the environment for years or even decades.

Almost all insecticides, herbicides, and chemical fertilizers are highly toxic, yet these products are widely used in commercial agriculture. Farmers are supposed to cease applying pesticides at regular times before harvesting. But few farmers with mortgage payments to meet will risk losing a crop. Some fruits are sprayed as many as fifteen times with carcinogenic pesticides.

Relatively few produce items on supermarket shelves are safe to eat without first being carefully peeled. The outer leaves of all leafy vegetables should be discarded and the rest washed. Many Hygienists refrain from eating commercially raised berries and grapes.

Yet toxic residues on fruits and vegetables are slight compared with those in meat, fish, and poultry. Although animal feed is no longer sprayed, studies show that meat, fish, and poultry contain 2-2½ times more pesticide residues than dairy products and 13 times more than fruits and vegetables. High fat animal foods, such as beef and cheese, show the highest levels of contamination while low fat products like yogurt and cottage cheese have least.

Fish, which live on smaller fish, which in turn feed on still smaller fish and organisms, build very high concentrations of toxic residues. Fish-eating birds like pelicans and ospreys—which are at the top of the food chain—have such a high concentration of pesticides and other toxins that many can no longer reproduce.

Another toxin used to fatten cattle is Diethylstilbestrol (DES), an estrogen. About twenty-five years ago, DES was given pregnant women to prevent miscarriages. Now some of the daughters of these women are developing unusually high rates of vaginal cancer. When this became known, the Department of Agriculture banned use of DES from animal feed not less than two weeks before slaughter. But residues of DES still remain in the livers of slaughtered animals.

People who eat fish, meat, and poultry are also eating high on the food chain. U.S. Government toxicity standards for pesticides and other food poisons are almost entirely based on short term tests on small animals. No consideration is given to such longterm effects as cancer or chronic liver damage.

The single worst environmental contamination known in history occurred during the mid-1970s when PBB (polybrominated biphenyl) was dumped into cattle feed by mistake at a Michigan chemical plant and was shipped to farmers all over the state. By 1977, almost nine million Michigan residents had been contaminated. As people consumed contaminated meat and dairy products and stored the PBB in their tissues, complaints of severe gastrointestinal disorders, liver abnormalities, nerve problems, severe headaches, swollen joints, loss of balance and hair, body rash, and rheumatoid arthritis were reported statewide.

Experts fear longterm cell damage, with cancer and genetic problems multiplying in future years. Yet Michigan Hygienists and other true vegetarians, all eating low on the food chain, escaped contamination altogether.

Wherever you live, the Hygienic way to safeguard yourself from ecologically concentrated pesticides and heavy metal poisoning is to eat low on the food chain. Animal fats, which carry the heaviest contamination, are

particularly high risk foods because they are also responsible for causing atherosclerosis.

Fried Foods and Fat Can Be Suicidal

So many studies have implicated a diet high in fats
and cholesterol with heart disease and several forms of
cancer that most nutritionists take the connection for
granted.

It's important to realize that not merely animal fats, but
all fats, increase the risk of heart disease. For years,
we've been told that unsaturated fats such as margarine
and vegetable oils were safe while butter and shortening
were not.

Not only is a high cholesterol level responsible for
atherosclerosis, but a high triglycerides (blood fats) level
can be even more damaging. A high triglycerides level is
caused by a high fat diet, even when the fat comes from
vegetable oils.

All fats and oils are doubly dangerous when heated for
they tend to become carcinogenic. In countries where
frying is common and fat is constantly re-heated,
stomach cancer is also common. Heated fat quickly becomes rancid and forms toxic peroxides. Because fat is
refrigerated in America and seldom re-used for frying,
stomach cancer rates in the U.S. have declined.

Unless preserved with anti-oxidants (also suspected of
being harmful to the human organism), vegetable oils—
including peanut butter—soon turn rancid and become
carcinogenic. Nowadays, most vegetable oils are also
highly processed and refined, treated with chemicals of
dubious safety, and often subjected to high heat and
pressure.

Anyone with the slightest regard for their health should
eliminate all vegetable oils and animal fats from their

30

diet immediately. Eating fried foods can be suicidal. If you *must* use vegetable oils, the safest are cold-pressed, unhydrogenated olive oil and safflower seed oil.

This caution is borne out by studies comparing the diet of Americans and Japanese. Forty-two percent of the average American diet consists of fat while only 10 percent of the average Japanese diet is fat. As might be expected, Japanese have only 10 percent of the heart disease found in Americans. A recent population survey also revealed that Japan had the lowest breast cancer rate in thirty-nine countries studied. When Japanese immigrate to the U.S., their heart disease rate becomes the same as for Americans.

Heart disease is also virtually unknown among the Bantu, the black people whose home is Southern Africa. Not surprisingly, the Bantu consume only 10 percent as much fat as Americans and their average cholesterol level is just 20 percent of ours. In 1975, only one American in ten had a serum cholesterol level under 200 mg. per cent. The Longevity Research Institute considers that any level over 160 causes artery damage.

Status and prestige are the reasons for our meat-centered diet. The more steak we consume, the higher we rate. To criticize steak, eggs, and dairy foods is still considered un-American (especially by the meat and dairy industries). Eggs have more cholesterol than any other food yet, on average, we consume 316 annually. Americans also eat half a pound of meat every day (thirty times the amount eaten by Japanese) and three-fourths of a pound of dairy products. While Americans have cut down somewhat on the use of eggs and high-fat dairy foods, consumption of meat rose twenty-six pounds per person during the past decade.

Studies by leading U.S., Canadian, and U.N. Nutritional organizations are unanimous in finding that the human organism normally requires a maximum of only .37 grams of animal protein or .51 grams of vegetable protein daily per pound of body weight. Thus a 130 pound woman requires about sixty-six grams of vegetable protein daily (under 2.5 ounces) and a 160 pound man about eight grams (about 2.75 ounces). Yet the average American consumes 157 grams of mostly meat protein—at least twice as much as the body can use. Protein cannot be stored in the body. It must be used immediatley and a fresh supply eaten daily.

A recent study in Colombia shows that the professional and managerial classes there consume three to thirty times as much beef as the poorer classes, nine times as much pork, six times as many eggs, five times as much milk, and eight time as much cooking oil. They also have four times as much bowel cancer and heart disease.

The number of studies linking an affluent diet high in fat and cholesterol with increased risk of cancer and heart disease are legion.

According to Dr. Ernst L. Wynder, President of the American Health Foundation, two of the biggest killers, cancer of the breast and colon, have been associated with affluent eating. Americans eat too much fat, says Dr. Wynder, 35-40 percent coming from meat. The body does not seem able to handle such high fat and cholesterol loads. In the case of colon cancer, a diet low in fiber and high in fats has been implicated. The typical American diet high in fat and cholesterol is the same one implicated as a major cause of heart disease.

The fat-rich foods that contain most cholesterol are shortening, lard, prime beef, hamburger, cured pork, seafoods, eggs, whole milk, chocolate, fatty cheeses, fried foods, and luncheon meat. Coconut is the only product of the vegetable kingdom to contain cholesterol. Coconut oil also contains cholesterol as do partially hydrogenated vegetable oils.

Curiously, only twenty-three percent of the diet of primitive Eskimo is comprised of fat. Wild animals and game are much leaner than feed lot-raised livestock. Not only are feed lot animals endangered by DES and possibly other hormones, but these animals are also routinely fed antibiotics as a prophylactic against disease. The condition of being crowded shoulder-to-shoulder in feed lots filled with excretion causes such stress that the animals' resistance to disease breaks down. Virus and bacterial diseases spread like wildfire.

Beef cattle are force-fed with sophisticated processed foods for 120-150 days before slaughter. This is because USDA beef grading is based on the proportion of marbled fat in meat. Choice-grade beef contains about sixty percent more fat than standard-grade meat. By making it more profitable to produce marbled beef than lean meat, the U.S. Government has been indirectly responsible for killing more Americans than have died in all the wars in which this country has participated since its origin.

Most cattle, pigs and chickens used to produce meat, eggs and dairy produce are far from healthy. Anyone who eats prime white veal should know that, to produce it, calves are confined in tiny windowless stalls and force-fed on a diet of high fat, artificial milk. According to the Coop Extension Service at the University of Massachusetts, veal calves become weak, anemic, and susceptible to disease. They frequently suffer from fungus infections, pneumonia, dysentery and diarrhea. Despite routine doses of wide spectrum antibiotics, as many as

10 percent die during confinement.

Most hogs are raised under equally artificial conditions, which accounts for the soft, pallid, and watery condition of most of today's hams.

Both eggs and chickens are frequently treated with antibiotics, and chickens are given anti-thyroid drugs and hormones. To stimulate more weight gain from less feed, chickens are raised on factory farms where they are confined in tiny assembly-line cages and fed by machines. Contagious disease runs rampant, and the birds are neurotic and disease-prone. Cirrhotic livers are common. As a result, eggs are pale, lacking in flavor and of poor quality. Chicken flesh is limp, comparatively tasteless and bloated with watery tissue.

Milk cows are also often confined in assembly line stalls and given hormones. The cows are purposely bred with udders so disproportionately large that many cows cannot consume enough food to support milk production. They frequently succumb to diseases like milk fever and swollen udders.

If you're thinking of powdered milk or non-dairy creamers as safe alternatives, consider this. Much of the nutritional value of powdered milk is lost by overprocessing and overheating. And non-dairy creamers are made from coconut oil, which can increase blood cholesterol levels as much as whole milk.

Undoubtedly, low-fat or no-fat dairy foods do offer complete protein with a minimum of fat. But like meat and all other animal-derived foods they lack any fiber and are the cause of hard stools. In view of the numerous risk factors so far described, Hygienists do not consider any kind of commercially produced meat, fish, poultry, seafood, eggs, or dairy foods acceptable for human consumption.

The Gremlins In Our Food   2002835

Today, foods are often preserved on supermarket shelves for months on end. Hundreds of different chemicals are added to make them prettier, better tasting, more convenient to prepare, longer lasting, and more profitable. But by extending shelf life, food manufacturers may be shortening the lives of consumers.

Every year, the average American consumes over four pounds of food additives. Among the most common are anti-oxidants, emulsifiers, stabilizers, bleaching agents, texturing agents, and nitrates. Flavoring agents are also frequently used to mask disagreeable flavors as well as to add artificial taste. Much commercial "whole wheat" bread is simply white bread with some whole wheat flour added plus some caramel coloring to turn the whole loaf a sickly, artificial brown. Texturing agents are used to make canned vegetables appear crisp and firm. Even fresh fruits and vegetables are often treated by supermarkets or their suppliers with fungicides, dyes, waxes, and pesticides. This is why all supermarket fruits and vegetables must be peeled or have their outer leaves removed.

How safe are these additives? Most Americans fondly imagine that the FDA is safeguarding their health. Not so! Through a "gentleman's agreement," the FDA expects the food industry to determine the safety of any new additives. Additives considered reasonably safe are classified as GRAS (Generally Recognized As Safe). But new additives are tested by feeding them to lab animals to determine how much it takes to kill half the animals in from one to fourteen days. The result is the Lethal Dose for 50 percent. No long term testing for cancer, mutation, or birth defects is made, nor is any consideration given to the risk of additive synergy—mixing one additive with another.

Under prodding by consumer groups, the FDA finally banned such additives as cyclamates, Red Dyes #2 and #4, butter yellow, Green #1, Orange #1 and #2, and carbon black. Red Dye #4, used primarily to color maraschino cherries, was suspected of causing urinary bladder polyps and shriveling the adrenal glands.

Yet almost 3,000 other additives remain in use. USE.

Among the most common is Monosodium Glutamate (MSG), commonly found in convenience foods, canned soups, meat, meat tenderizers, fish fillets, salad dressings, poultry, candy, and Chinese restaurants. Brain lesions have been found in infant animals fed doses of MSG equivalent in magnitude to those used in food. Manufacturers have now removed MSG from baby foods. But it is still common in Italian and Oriental restaurants and in numerous varieties of supermarket foods.

Nitrates and nitrites, used in curing and smoking meats, fish, bacon, luncheon meats, corned beef, canned ham, and sausage have been found to produce nitrosamines when eaten. Nitrosamines are considered the most prevalent diet-associated carcinogen in the U.S. Fried bacon is a common source of nitrosamines.

Even peanuts and Brazil nuts are treated with a mould-inhibitor to retard aflatoxin, another very dangerous carcinogen which appears in peanuts when improperly stored.

Salt is another additive we could all do without. It is a direct cause of high blood pressure and Americans use four times as much per capita as the remainder of the human race. The slight trace required for human nutrition is adequately supplied by fruits and vegetables. An apple, for instance, contains 1 mg. of salt. But a hamburger contains over 500 mgs., and processed cheese is equally high in sodium.

Food containers are treated with chemicals of unknown toxicity. Paperboard containers are coated with waxes and polymeric resins while metal containers are often coated with resins or lacquers. All may rub off on food. Plastic used for wrapping cold cuts contain chemicals believed to harm the body and vinyl chloride is reported to leach from plastic containers into food.

In the average large supermarket today, it is virtually impossible to find more than two or three items which have not been contaminated with additives or treated with some kind of chemical. Big food conglomerates have launched huge publicity offensives to convince the public that additives are essential and that without them, food costs would soar.

None of which worries Hygienists very much. By using only fresh, living vegetarian foods, Hygienists eliminate the whole litany of risks associated with eating embalmed, processed foods and foods of animal origin. By carefully peeling or removing the outer leaves of all commercially raised fruit and produce, Hygienists are able to reduce contamination to only a tiny fraction of that which threatens non-vegetarians.

The Grim Effects of Counterfeit Foods

Every year, Americans flush 1240 millions worth of

constipation remedies down the toilet, all due to eating a low residue diet of animal-derived foods and highly refined carbohydrates. By comparison, the average Hygienist typically has two or three impromptu bowel movements daily and passes soft, bulky stools which yield easily without ever causing difficulty or discomfort. Hygienists do not keep reading material in the bathroom. The whole process is over in well under a minute.

The unfailing regularity of Hygienists is due, of course, to the extremely high fiber content of the Hygienic diet. Hygienists live almost exclusively on fresh uncooked fruits, vegetables, nuts, and seeds. They do not need bran.

British researcher Dr. Dennis Burkett, who has studied bowel cancer in Africans, believes that the high colon cancer rates in the U.S., and England are due to the large quantity of refined grains and cereals eaten and to the predominance of low residue meat, eggs and dairy foods in the diet. Burkett found that in East Africa, where people eat large amounts of unrefined cereals and grains, colon cancer rates are extremely low. He believes that fiber sweeps out food wastes that otherwise accumulate in the colon and that encourage the growth of bacteria which produce carcinogens.

Grains and cereals are refined to make them last longer on supermarket shelves. Refining destroys the germ of the grain and removes almost all fiber. In the process, almost all vitamins and minerals are leached out, leaving only empty calories. The highly refined American diet has been linked with an increasing risk of cancer of the lower intestines, appendicitis, risk of intestinal blockage, and atherosclerosis.

The most common refined carbohydrates are white

sugar, white flour, white bread, and white rice.

Including sugar in syrups and processed foods, the average American consumes 125 pounds of white sugar annually. Recent studies have implicated sugar as causing a variety of ailments from diabetes to obesity, high blood pressure, fatty liver, heart disease, and duodenal ulcers. Some researchers have suggested that a sugar-free diet will increase your lifespan.

Eliminating sugar doesn't mean you just stop buying sugar. Almost all canned, processed, and convenience foods are larded with it. Sugar is also extensively used in pasta, breads, chow mein, blue cheese, sauces, pickles, soda drinks, fried rice mixtures, cakes and pastries, candy, and breakfast cereals. Nearly 50 percent of some children's breakfast cereal consists of white sugar.

According to eminent nutritionist Dr. Jean Mayer, the human body requires no sugar at all. Sugar contains no vitamins, minerals, protein or other nutrients, merely hollow calories that cause millions of dental cavities each year. Hygienists concur wholeheartedly with Dr. Mayer and also believe that brown sugar, honey, and molasses are no better. The Hygienic diet is completely free of sweeteners of any type.

Milling white flour from whole grain removes almost all of the vitamins B1, B2, E, and Niacin as well as most of the calcium, phosphorus, iron, and potassium. Bakers replace some, but not all, of these losses by enriching white bread with synthetic vitamins. But they cannot replace the fiber. The average American factory-made loaf is as limp as a wad of cotton and tastes like Kleenex.

In college towns and larger cities, unrefined breads and cereals are now available at natural food stores and graineries. But such items as wheat germ, unprocessed rolled oats, or genuine whole wheat or sourdough bread, are often impossible to find in smaller towns.

Again, Hygienists are entirely unaffected by the spectre of food refining. For though Hygienists may occasionally eat whole-grain breads or cereals when traveling or backpacking, these acid-forming foods are not a regular part of the Hygienic diet.

Stimulants are Life Destroying

Alcohol, not heroin, is the most abused drug in America and well over half our adult population is hooked on such narcotics as alcohol, cigarettes, and coffee.

Smoking and its effects kill a thousand people a day in the U.S. Over 2,000 separate studies have proved that, whether from cigarettes, pipe, or cigar, nicotine attacks heart, lungs, and brain and has killed more people than all the great epidemics of the last hundred years put together. Anyone who continues to smoke is committing a slow but inevitable form of suicide that invariably leads to death and destruction.

Some studies claim to have shown that, by a slight margin, elderly people who drink very moderately tend to outlive those who don't. However, half of all Americans who have reached ninety have never tasted alcohol. The fact remains that alcohol is a drug that depresses the central nervous system, increases pulse rate, and inhibits the function of the heart muscle and liver. A 1976 study by the National Institutes of Health showed that regular alcohol consumption increases risk of breast cancer in women by 20-60 percent, of thyroid cancer in both men and women by 30-150 percent, and of skin cancer by 20-70 percent. The more one drinks, the greater the risk.

Other studies have linked drinking with bladder cancer and with birth defects caused by both mother *and* father. A single night of heavy drinking can cause aberrations in a man's sperm cells that may result in serious birth defects in an offspring. The fact that one American child in fourteen is born with a birth defect is undoubtedly due, in part, to the widespread drinking habits of American males.

Coffee is nothing but a legal shot of speed so potent that it constricts the blood vessels in the brain and dilates them elsewhere throughout the body. A single cup will allay fatigue and drowsiness and pep up the thought process. Several cups will accelerate the pulse, increase blood pressure, raise free fatty acid levels, and interfere with sleep. Yet the average American adult drinks at least three cups per day.

Dr. Hershel Jick and Dr. Dennis Slone, working on a drug surveillance program at Boston University, found that by drinking six cups per day, risk of heart attack is increased by an estimated 120 percent. For people who drink only one to five cups per day, the risk is still increased by 60 percent. According to Dr. Philip T. Cole of Harvard University School of Public Health, women who drink at least one cup per day may incur a risk of bladder cancer 250 percent greater than non-caffeine drinking women. (In men, the risk is only increased by 25 percent.) Other studies show that pregnant women who drink caffeine—whether in coffee, tea, cola drinks, cocoa, or chocolate—run a greatly increased risk of miscarriage, stillbirth, or fetal death.

A cup of brewed coffee contains approximatley 80

mgs. of caffeine. Instant coffee contains slightly less. A ten-ounce cola drink has 40 mg. of caffeine, a cup of cocoa 42 mg., and a cup of leaf tea 45 mg. Pharmacologists consider a dose larger than 250 mg. as "large." This is just three cups—a single hour's ration for many coffee habitués. Such excessive coffee drinking can produce symptoms identical to those of anxiety, irritability, rapid breathing, and heart fibrillation. On all too many occasions, American doctors suspect that they are being asked to prescribe tranquillizers for nothing more than coffee overdose.

Decaffeinated coffee isn't much better. Although a cup contains only two mg. of caffeine, according to Ralph Nader's Health Research Group, a chemical called Trichloroethylene (TCE) used in some brands has produced cancer in lab animals.

Through a short fast, Natural Hygiene offers the surest and quickest method for permanently eliminating all of these life-threatening stimulants.

Even The Water Isn't Safe

Evidence isn't conclusive yet but many scientists suspect a strong correlation between cancer of the urinary organs and organic chemicals in drinking water across the U.S.

Nowadays, ground waters are frequently polluted by nitrates and nitrites from agricultural fertilizers. The human organism readily converts these into nitrosamines, one of the most potent carcinogens known.

Every year, over 3.5 billion tons of waste and garbage is disposed of, much of which eventually ends up in U.S. water supplies. Chlorine is added to purify the water. But chlorine reacts with organic compounds in water to form chloroform. A 1975 survey of drinking water in eight U.S. cities by the EPA found chloroform the most common contaminant. The EPA study also found that death rates from gastrointestinal and urinary tract cancer was 44 percent higher among people who drank chlorinated water than in populations drinking untreated water.

No amount of chlorine can screen out such metallic pollutants as lead, asbestos, cadmium, aluminum, silver, and titanium, all found in various U.S. water supplies and able to cause high blood pressure and cancer, among other things.

To make matters worse, dentists and others have convinced well-meaning city governments to add fluoride to drinking water to prevent cavities in children's teeth. In 1970, the National Cancer Society warned of increasing cancer death rates in populations drinking artificially fluoridated water. Five years later, the impressive studies of Dr. John Yiamouyouiannis, Science Director of the National Health Federation, and Dr. Dean Burk, a founder of the National Cancer Institute, showed conclusively that in cities which fluoridated their water, cancer death rates rose by 5-15 percent. The Yiamouyouiannis-Burk studies revealed sharp increases in cancer of the gastrointestinal tract starting two to five years after fluoride is first introduced into drinking water.

Another study by Dr. Ionel Rapaport at the University of Wisconsin showed that mongolism in infants increased in direct proportion to the amount of fluoride added to water. The various studies also showed that 1 p.p.m. parts per million of sodium fluoride added to water interferes with bone growth, nerve functions, the endocrine gland system, and tends to promote kidney stones. Yet cities all over America continue to add fluoride to drinking water at the rate of 1-1.4 p.p.m.

Today, many scientists tend to believe that unless you live in a remote area where your water is uncontaminated by industry, agriculture or water plant treatment, your drinking water is probably carcinogenic.

There are several possible solutions: 1. go out once a month and fill about twenty-five one-gallon glass jugs with pure water from an uncontaminated source such as a well, spring, or mountain stream; 2. buy bottled water; or 3. buy a stainless steel (not aluminum) water distiller and distill your own 100 percent pure water. Failing these, you can remove most of the chlorine and chloroform from water by boiling it for at least three minutes before drinking. However, though initially more expensive, over the long run the third alternative will prove to be the safest and cheapest method.

Our Poisoned Environment

We're living and working among a minefield of cancer causing agents. Some jobs in manufacturing plants must be closed to pregnant women because chemicals may cause fetus damage. But nothing is done to safeguard non-pregnant women and men working on these same jobs.

Any job in which you come into contact with asbestos, lead, chromates, analine dyes, vinyl chloride, or similar toxins may be a short cut to cancer of the lung or bladder. About ten million American workers who handle asbestos run a risk of dying of lung cancer seven to ten times greater than the general population. The risk also extends to their families.

So much fresh evidence of increasing risk due to carcinogenic chemicals keeps emerging that the EPA must constantly set new regulations limiting exposure. Over 4.6 million Americans live within five miles of plants making or processing vinyl chloride, and evidence suggests that they, too, are exposed to a more than normal risk. So polluted are many of our cities that breathing the air involves the same risk as smoking several cigarettes per day. Constant low-level exposure to polluted air can lead to a whole alphabet of ailments. Approximately 20 percent of all lung cancer, respiratory diseases, bronchitis, and emphysema is directly caused by polluted air. Breathing the air in our big cities for even half a day impairs the ability of the blood to carry oxygen to the brain and causes irritability and a run-down feeling.

Cosmetics and hair dyes are just one example of many ways in which we can be intoxicated by heavy metal poisoning. According to a report by Dr. Robert C. Lynch, Director of the Preventative Medical Clinic of Downer's Grove, Ill., a number of hair dyes and cosmetics contain toxic levels of copper, zinc, mercury, or lead. The metals are most common in brush-in or comb-in hair dyes and in many popular cosmetics ranging from face powder to eye shadow, shampoo, and hair sprays. The metals are easily absorbed through the skin, causing nervousness, depression, insomnia, anxiety, listlessness, and mood swings.

Noise is another form of pollution that can raise blood pressure, heighten nervousness and tension, increase susceptibility to infection, and even raise fat and cholesterol levels. The EPA reports that noise levels in U.S. cities have been doubling every ten years. Today, the average noise level in urban environments is eighty-five decibels, the maximum considered safe for human ears.

The agency considers that noise pollution poses a serious hazard for approximately forty million Americans. *Consumer Reports* magazine (October 1975) also maintains that the number of Americans suffering from hearing loss will grow as noise levels escalate. Many experts believe that deafness in the aged is merely the result of long term exposure to low level sound.

The extent of hearing damage depends not only on the sound level but on the duration of exposure. One way to block out noise and thereby allow the ear to recover is to wear a plastic hearing protector. But many Hygienists, as well as tens of thousands of other Americans, have felt that a better remedy is too simply move away from big city noise and pollution if possible.

Radiation—The Silent Killer

Only twenty years ago, some experts claimed that exposure to 1,000 rads of radiation per year was a safe level for workers in nuclear installations. Subsequent experience showed that the minimum exposure which could cause cancer was far lower. The current permissible level is five rads per year. Even this is too high according to Dr. Irwin D. J. Bross of Roswell Park Memorial Institute in Buffalo, N.Y. Dr. Bross believes that levels below five rads can produce an increased risk of leukemia in a person exposed to radiation, as well as in their offspring. No one knows exactly what minimum level is entirely safe. A smaller dosage simply means it will take longer for cancer to appear.

That is why we must be exceptionally careful to avoid unnecessary exposure to diagnostic X-rays. A full mouth dental X-ray can produce an exposure of approximately 2.5 rads, a mammography—used to detect breast cancer—from 1 to 3 rads.

46

Because repeated doses of X-rays over a long period may cause more cancers than they help to diagnose, the National Cancer Institute in 1976 ceased to recommend routine mammography screening of healthy women under fifty. For every rad of X-ray dosage, the risk of breast cancer is increased by 1 percent or more. One year later, the Institute reported that 29-100 percent of women under fifty were still receiving mammography— indicative of how the medical profession continually endangers its patients by disregarding guidelines.

Exposure to radiation is cumulative for life and we are constantly being exposed to low-level radiation from such sources as microwave ovens, color TV sets, and fluorescent lights. Here again, however, the Hygienic lifesyle has eliminated any need for microwave ovens. Through cutting out sugar and refined carbohydrates, most Hygienists enjoy such improved dental health that X-rays are seldom required. Many Hygienists prefer to do something more constructive than to watch TV. And as I write this book, my fluorescent lampholder is still overhead but has been minus tubes for several years. Instead, I have three 100-watt bulbs strung on it.

We're Playing Russian Roulette With Our Lives

Things people do are a major cause of toxemia. Broiling meat over a backyard charcoal burner, for instance, produces benzopyrene, a known carcinogen, in the meat. The Pill has enabled millions of people to engage in sex without worrying about birth control. But the Pill itself is a suspected carcinogen and gonorrhea has reached epidemic proportions. Several studies indicate that 5-10 percent of all young American women have gonorrhea. In 1976 a new penicillin-resistant strain from the Philippines spread to the U.S. (the Center for

Disease Control in Atlanta fears this may become the dominant type of gonorrhea). Over a million Americans become infected with gonorrhea annually. Another widespread veneral disease is Herpes Simplex Virus II, which has been linked to cervical cancer in women.

Millions more Americans, in their desire to achieve, develop competitive, aggressive personalities that lead to stress. What they are trying to achieve is to earn more money to buy more things that, in the final analysis, are bad for their health. The lives of millions of men and women is pressured to meet deadlines and time requirements. As an antidote to the frantic pace, people eat, drink and smoke more, and pop tranquilizers.

Stress is a shapeless cause of toxemia, but its symptoms are always the same: ulcers, colitis, high blood pressure, and heart attack. Yet the most perilous effect of stress is its debilitating effect on the immune system, weakening the body's defenses against cancer, arthritis, multiple sclerosis, and infectious diseases like pneumonia.

Vigorous physical exercise is the best antidote to stress. Yet most people still exert themselves as little as possible. Rather than shovel snow or cut grass with a hand mower, they buy power driven machines which only aggravate their need to earn still more money. Not only do machines rob us of essential exercise but frequently break down, require constant searching for spare parts, and many are ineffective in what they are claimed to do.

As a society, we are obsessively concerned with eating. Approximately one American in four is overweight and many people in their twenties and thirties are already obese. The average American eats almost three times as much as the average Vilcabamban and gets about one tenth as much exercise. Millions of Americans have middle-aged bodies by age thirty-five.

The Abkhasians consider a fat person sick. The Mayo Clinic also regards obesity as a disease. And for good reason. Obese people run a greatly increased risk of angina and heart disease, nephritis, gall bladder problems, diabetes, cirrhosis of the liver, respiratory disorders, and hernias. Self-caused diseases are virtually unknown to anyone who faithfully follows the Hygienic lifestyle.

If reading this chapter gives you a Doomsday feeling, you are not alone. Many eminent scientists belive that our planet is so poisoned that human life cannot endure for another hundred years. At a 1976 meeting of the American Association for the Advancement of Science in Boston, a writer asked Virginia L. Zaratzan, Ph.D., a pharmacologist with the National Institute of Health, if the human race was doomed.

"Yes, absolutely," Dr. Zaratzian replied. She is convinced that unless potentially harmful chemicals are removed from our food, air, and water, the human race faces a soaring cancer risk.

We are living in such a perilously chemicalized society that only by studiously avoiding every one of the health-destroying factors described in this chapter, can we hope to survive and live out our full natural lifespan in robust good health.

No other health care system is so totally suited to safeguard our health against the worldwide peril of chemical overkill as Natural Hygiene. Based entirely on living in harmony with Nature, Natural Hygiene offers a disease-free lifestyle which literally eliminates every one of the toxemia-producing factors profiled in his chapter.

3

Why Americans Don't Get Well
The Over-medicated Society

Brenda H., was only twenty-nine when her doctor diagnosed ulcerative colitis. She was immediately placed on several different drugs, including tranquilizers and antibiotics, and forbidden to eat fatty meats, eggs, or raw foods.

A year later, Brenda was rushed to hospital suffering from adverse drug reactions. A specialist prescribed more drugs and put her back on fatty meats, eggs, and raw foods. Gradually, her sight deteriorated, she lost twenty pounds and developed hemorrhoids.

In desperation, Brenda tried another doctor. She was immediately sent to hospital and given massive amounts of cortisone, pencillin, and tranquilizers. Altogether, during her illness, thirty-eight different drugs were prescribed. Approximately half the drugs were to offset the side effects of other drugs.

Next, Brenda came down with cortisone poisoning. She developed an enlarged abdomen, a moon face, and muscle spasms. Each day, she had at least twenty bowel movements and was unable to travel or enjoy any family life. Her hemorrhoids became gangrenous and had to be cut out. The doctor advised Brenda to have her colon removed and to move her bowels into a plastic bag hooked to her waist. Meanwhile, a new set of grapevine hemorrhoids appeared.

At this stage, six years after her illness began, a friend recommended Natural hygiene. When Brenda first applied for admission to a Hygienic institution, she was turned down because of the excessive toxemia created by her prolonged medication. But finally she was accepted.

Weak and emaciated, she was placed on a fast. By the ninth day, her colitis symptoms had disappeared. After thirty-three more days without eating, her hemorrhoids also disappeared. Brenda broke her fast on the forty-second day and has not had colitis or any other ailment since.

Today, ten years later, Brenda still has her colon and exudes good health and vitality. Each year, she takes a therapeutic fast and each year she reaches a new plateau of health and well being.

Brenda is one of thousands of Americans who, thoroughly disillusioned by orthodox medical treatment, have finally sought to recover their health through more natural and holistic therapies. Although Natural Hygiene is not strictly a therapy, it is one of a group of closely related, totally natural health care systems that include hatha yoga, Arica, biological medicine, and the lifestyle of the Seventh Day Adventists.

As more and more Americans become disenchanted

51

with the disappointing results and high costs of old style orthodox medical care, they are turning to alternative therapies in ever increasing numbers. Today the holistic health movement is growing at an unprecedented pace. The natural approach to getting well is scoring such fantastic gains that even some doctors are becoming concerned by the lack of success of medical treatment. Already, small groups of doctors are beginning to form health care organizations with such titles as "New Lifestyle" or "Prevention."

Instead of cutting out organs, these doctors cut out causes of disease. They use only natural methods that create no side effects, leave no scarring or disability, and they charge a fraction of the price of current medical care.

But the main thrust of the holistic health movement is being led not by doctors but by Natural Hygienists, yogis, Vegans, Preventionists, chiropractors, physical therapists, and natural food enthusiasts. The movement has gained such momentum that even highly placed physicians are becoming disturbed at the estrangement that is rapidly developing between the American public and the medical profession.

Dr. Walter McNerney, President of the Blue Cross Association, was quoted in 1976 as saying that he believes the U.S. is wasting billions annually by concentrating on research areas that offer relatively minor possibilities of improvement and on the development of exotic equipment and hospitals. Dr. McNerney said it was increasingly evident that betterment of national health and wellbeing is to be found in the study of the environment, lifestyle, and culture from which so many modern ailments arise. He recommended a holistic approach rather than the current fragmented emphasis on only isolated aspects of health.

The medical establishment today consists of a huge drug industry; about 400,000 physicians; thousands of hospitals and clinics; and armies of cashiers, nurses, pharmacists, technicians, and secretaries, all depending for their livelihood on medical treatment. In 1975, the U.S. spent $118 billions on medical care. Yet in 1976, there was more heart disease, cancer, and arthritis than ever.

These disappointing results occur because a lot of medical treatment simply doesn't work. Medicine's greatest triumphs are in dealing with crisis and emergencies and in treating injuries and burns. In treating disease, allopathy's record is something less than convincing. A lot of treatment doesn't work because instead of treating the patient holistically, doctors have chosen to become specialists in such fragmented areas as diseases of the thoracic cavity, digestive system, or eyes, ears, nose, and throat.

Something like 70 percent of all human ailments are self-limiting or eventually clear up of their own accord. The overall healing rate of allopathy is also about 70 percent. This would seem to indicate that people might get well just as readily by not consulting a physician. If this is true, it is because doctors of medicine are trained to use drugs and surgery instead of the body's own healing powers.

Many Mutilating Operations Are Actually Unnecessary

During 1975-76 hearings of the House Oversight and Investigative Subcommittee headed by California Congressman John E. Moss, the committee learned that in

1974, doctors performed approximately 2,800,000 unnecessary operations cauing 11,900 needless deaths. Based on a review of medical literature, studies done under Government contract, and information from hospitals, it was estimated that 220,000 hysterectomies and 130,000 tonsillectomies were unnecessarily performed and that the public paid approximately $4 billions for operations they didn't need.

While this was going on, a committee sponsored by the American College of Surgeons and the American Surgical Association concluded a five year study by announcing in 1975 that the U.S. has about 30,000 more surgeons than it needs. The study found 94,000 doctors practicing surgery in the U.S., while the nation's needs could readily be met by only 52,000 board-certified surgeons.

Doctors sometimes turn to surgery instead of general practice because surgery is more profitable To consult a surgeon is an open invitation to be told you need an expensive operation. Surgeons obtain their income by practicing surgery, not by recommending exercise or diet. In Great Britain, which has only half as many surgeons per capita as the U.S., the number of operations done is also exactly half as many per capita as in the U.S. Yet British health and longevity standards are actually slightly better than in America.

Cutting out organs, such as gallbladders or tonsils, impairs the function of the whole body. Everything in the body contributes a necessary role. Circumcision has been severly criticized by the American Academy of Pediatricians; and vasectomized men have been found to undergo a hormonal change. Over the years, tens of millions of children have had their tonsils removed on medical advice in order to prevent colds. But investigations have shown that removing tonsils tends to *increase* susceptibility to colds. Tonsils also play a role in the immunological system, and removal may create a predisposition to cancer later in life.

In his book, *The Solid Gold Stethoscope,* published in 1976, Dr. Edgar Berman, Senator Hubert Humphrey's personal physician, concludes that fewer than 15 percent of all American doctors are really hard working and dedicated to their patients. Too many, he says, are more dedicated to the dollar.

Social commentator Ivan Illich, in his recent book *Medical Nemesis: the Expropriation of Health,* also points out that statistics tend to show that the more health care there is, the shorter the life expectancy.

Despite all the triumphs of medical science, in 1976 an American male aged sixty had a life expectancy only two years longer than in 1789. In twenty-five other countries, including Greece, Italy, Bulgaria, Poland, and Hungary, men live longer than they do in America. In these countries, men receive far less medical care and medication than we do.

Advances in nutrition have not been incorporated into medical education. For years, the American Diabetes and American Dietetic Associations have been urging doctors to treat diabetics with a low-fat, high-carbohydrate diet in place of drugs and insulin. Though this diet is medically endorsed, relatively few doctors are aware of this development, and most new diabetics are still put on insulin and drugs.

Only a dozen or so medical schools in the U.S., have departments of nutrition. Yet studies have shown that 80 percent of all human ailments are directly attributable to diet. Many doctors are still treating nutritional deficiencies with drugs. Several investigations have revealed that laymen are often better informed about health and nutrition than their physicians.

Authorities estimate that about 15,000 American doctors are actually incompetent. One surgeon, for example, read an X-ray of a woman's kidneys backwards and cut out the healthy kidney, leaving the woman with only a cancerous one. Hospitals ask incompetent doctors to resign, but state medical societies almost never revoke a fellow physician's license, and these doctors continue to practice. Medical malpractice suits are reaching crisis proportions as people lose faith in medical science and lose confidence in their physicians.

A Nation Of Junkies

A pill for every ill is the message of many TV commercials. Through medical propaganda and the scare ads of drug companies, Americans are taking prescription and non-prescription drugs on a massive scale. Thousands of drugs are used not only to treat serious diseases but for headaches, sleeplessness, indigestion, to make women look younger, to prevent conception, to lose weight, and for almost every minor ache, discomfort, inconvenience, and social annoyance.

Women who are distressed by the routine of household chores are saturated with psychoactive drugs like tranquilizers. Psychotropic drugs are widely used to combat mood changes and to affect our behavior.

According to the World Health Organization, 47.5 percent of the American populace is on some type of medication. Both adults and children are becoming a nation of junkies.

In elementary schools, an estimated two million children are being given drugs to counteract hyperactivity. Prior to 1965, hyperactivity was unheard of. Unless children take the daily doses prescribed, principals threaten to keep them out of school. So widespread is the drugging of schoolchildren and so frightening are the side effects—children retarded in height and weight growth and turned into docile vegetables—that angry parents have formed organizations to combat it. Many parents claim that drugging is merely a convenient way to make large classes easier for teachers to handle.

Hygienic children do not have hyperactive behavioral or learning problems. The work of Dr. Ben F. Feingold of the Kaiser Permanente Medical Center in San Francisco shows that hyperactivity in children is directly related to additives in supermarket foods. Children who were changed over to an additive-free diet soon lost all hyperactive symptoms.

Older persons, too, are so frequently overdrugged that they become spaced-out and disoriented. Dr. K. Warren Schale, Director of the University of California's Gerontology Research Institute, found that outside institutions, 25 percent of elderly persons considered senile were simply disoriented by misused drugs. Among long-term residents of nursing homes, Dr. Schale found that one in two persons were actually suffering drug-induced disorientation that could easily be reversed.

The drugging of both young and old is a heartbreaking human tragedy. Not only are all drugs toxic, but through insidious advertising the drug companies are promoting dependency for life on many drugs which have not been adequately tested for long term effects.

"Every medication is a double edged sword," writes

Joe Graedon in his best selling book *The Peoples' Pharmacy.* "Successful treatment is a balance between the beneficial and harmful effects hopefully weighted in favor of the beneficial."

Over a billion drug prescriptions are written annually by U.S. physicians and every year, 1.5 million people are admitted to U.S. hospitals with Adverse Drug Reactions (ADRs). Not infrequently, drug medications cause such awesome side effects as dizziness, nausea, fever, rash, stomach cramps, loss of balance, itching, blurred vision, loss of appetite, joint pains, insomnia, fluttering, constipation, depression, drowsiness, and impotence. Adverse side effects from prescription drugs are so common that in 1976 Grosset & Dunlap published *Prescription Drugs and Their Side Effects,* a guide to the side effects of 150 common medications.

Man-Made Diseases Are Shortening Our Lives

Harsh and dangerous drugs not only produce temporary side effects of varying intensity but in some cases, they can create iatrogenic diseases that can be as bad as the condition they are claimed to cure. An iatrogenic disease is a drug- or doctor-caused disease, and one study recently showed that iatrogenic diseases are so widespread that they are now ranked as the eleventh cause of death in the U.S.

Every drug presents two undeniable risks: **1.** It may not remedy or benefit the condition for which it is prescribed. **2.** It is toxic and can only increase the underlying condition of toxemia which is responsible for the very disease the drug is being prescribed to help.

Antibiotics, for example, do kill bacteria. But along with infectious invading organisms, they also annihilate friendly bacteria that are an essential part of the digestive

58

process. Originally, antibiotics were reserved for severe cases of pneumonia, meningitis, and venereal disease. Today they are frequently prescribed for such mild complaints as the common cold—against which they are totally ineffective.

The more drugs and medical treatment that science produces, the larger becomes the army of sick and disabled people. As medical facilities proliferate, overall health standards deteriorate. Almost every week, some new drug is introduced with great fanfare as the final panacea for one or more diseases. Six months later, it is completely forgotten. The side effects were too harsh or the drug turned out to be less beneficial than believed. So the scramble continues for ever new and more powerful drugs—and the drugging goes on and on.

Here's how Dr. Robert S. Mendelsohn, assistant Director of Michael Rees Hospital, Chicago, sees it: "From birth to death, we live in an over-medicated society. Rest assured that if there's not a pill now available designed to cure what ails you, someone's working on one. And just as surely, there's going to be something about the pill that's potentially hazardous to your health."

The totally unholistic concept of allopathy has encouraged the proliferation of specialists of all kinds of medical practice. Instead of healing the whole person, a patient goes to one doctor for heart trouble, another doctor for digestive problems, another doctor for respiratory ailments. Frequently, patients do not tell each doctor what another physician has already prescribed and on the basis of one drug for each disease, each doctor prescribes a different medication. The result is a therapeutic cocktail that often has devastating effects.

Doctors also frequently prescribe additional drugs to treat the side effects of drugs already being used. Addi-

59

tional drugs may then be needed to treat the side effects of the new drugs and so on, *ad infinitum*. In the 1950s and 1960s, there was massive prescribing of combinations of antibiotics like penicillin and streptomycin. This overuse created strains of antibiotic-resistant bacteria which still infect millions of patients every year in hospitals and which have threatened worldwide epidemics.

The Establishment Is On A Collison Course With Health

Physicians are not entirely responsible for the widespread abuse of drugs. Doctors are under tremendous pressure from drug companies and manufacturers of sophisticated medical equipment to use "cures" that are profitable to these companies.

Every year, for example, Congress votes $600 millions for cancer research. Almost all of this is spent on seeking cures that would be profitable to manufacturers of drug and medical equipment. Huge sums are being spent to investigate a cure for virus-caused cancer although numerous studies show that 80-90 percent of all cancers are caused by environmental carcinogens. Other promising leads are totally ignored so that funds may be steered instead into the coffers of drug and hospital equipment companies. No wonder cancer is called "Medicine's Vietnam." In spite of the billions spent, the armies of scientists and their supporters on the payroll, there has been no major breakthrough nor any real progress in cancer treatment since the mid-1950s.

Conflicts of interest occur at every stage of medical treatment, from doctors who can profit by recommending expensive operations to employees of cancer organizations who have financial connections wih corporations that manufacture carcinogens. Drug manufacturers subsidize the very university medical labs which carry out "unbiased" tests on their drugs.

In early 1977, U.S. Representative Benjamin Rosenthal (D-NY) and consumer watchdog Dr. Michael Jacobson, warned that many of America's foremost university nutritionists and food doctors had vested interests in food corporations. The nutritionists frequently act as consultants to giant food corporations and testify on their behalf at Congressional hearings. Some university nutritionists sit on the boards of directors of large food manufacturing corporations.

Whenever you hear nutritionists staunchly defending sugar, refined foods, commercial breakfast cereals, or food additives, chances are high that their work is being funded by the food industry. According to Dr. Jacobson, Director of the non-profit Center for Science in the Public Interest, university departments of nutrition are ridden with corporate influence from food industry giants.

Whenever the FDA discovers a suspected carcinogen in a widely-used food or container, and attempts to have it banned, armies of lobbyists and lawyers descend on Washington to fight the decision.

Numerous employees of the FDA have complained that, whenever they oppose actions sought by drug companies, they were harassed and punished by their superiors. The reason given is that many high FDA officials eventually quit the agency for more lucrative jobs in drug companies. To do so, they must show an unblemished record of never having challenged drugs manufactured by the firm they hope to work for.

Immunizations Cause Toxemia

Hygienists consider that a healthy organization should

be able to quickly manufacture its own antibodies against infectious virus and bacteria. Immunizations are regarded as a threatening and unnecessary form of tox-emia. Hygienists do not accept immunizations of any kind and do not permit their children to be innoculated.

Infectious disease statistics support the Hygienic ar-gument. Most people, for instance, erroneously believe that through immunization, medical science has con-quered many diseases that were formerly pandemic. Granted, immunizations for polio, measles, and smallpox have been effective. But most of the decline in infectious diseases of childhood has been due to improved sanita-tion and nutrition, not to the triumphs of medical sci-ence.

For instance, the combined death rate for scarlet fever, diphtheria, whooping cough, and measles for children up to age fifteen in England and Wales between 1860 and 1965 shows that nearly 90 percent of the total decline occurred before the introduction of antibiotics and wide-spread immunization. Another study shows that in the U.S., infectious diseases of infancy and childhood, such as T.B., declined by 70 percent between 1900 and 1940. Antibiotics and widespread immunization were not available before 1940.

Hygienists are not alone in opposing immunizations. Millions of ordinary Americans became disenchanted with unrestricted immunizations when the U.S. Govern-ment introduced the swine flu vaccine in late 1976. The program became a fiasco when the vaccine was as-sociated with the Guillain-Barré syndrome, a rare form of paralysis.

Hygienists suspect that only those already debilitated by toxemia are hit by infectious diseases. People who eat and live healthfully are able to fight off infections. Thus Hygienists object to having a toxic condition created in their bodies by immunizations.

The average Hygienist believes that he cannot trust his health to the hands of the Government, the food or drug industries, or the medical profession.

Hygienists recall the thalidomide diaster, when children were born with gross body defects after the mothers took doctor-prescribed thalidomide. They recall how, in the 1920s, doctors advised millions of adults to have healthy teeth pulled out because they were a source of "focal" infection. "Focal" infection proved to be a giant myth. Hygienists feel that many doctors are still floundering around today, giving patients one drug after another in the desperate hope of finding a cure.

Hygienists feel that where safeguarding their health is concerned, they must rely entirely on themselves.

That is why Hygienists insist on exercising sovereign rights over their own bodies and why they assume complete responsibility for their own health. After reading these chapters it must be patently obvious why Hygienists tend to be almost entirely free of the ubiquitous toxemia that eventually causes fatal degenerative diseases in almost everyone else.

Natural Hygiene

Nature's Bombshell Therapy for Most Human Ailments

Shortly after his marriage, Ted E. started getting colds and indigestion. Only 30 years old, he felt constantly tired.

Like many other young people, Ted and his wife enjoyed exotic foods and wines, and both smoked a pack or more of cigarettes a day. But soon pain appeared in Ted's hands and in joints all over his body. Before long, his knees became swollen and his fingers looked like sausages. Ted's neck was so still that bending became an ordeal. Ted's physician diagnosed his condition as rheumatoid arthritis and said there was no cure.

He prescribed aspirin six times daily. The aspirin caused a rash on Ted's chest and arms. The doctor then prescribed anti-histamine for the rash. He also gave Ted cortisone.

The cortisone upset Ted's digestion. Other disturbing

side effects appeared. Finally, Ted was sent to hospital. During his six-weeks stay, he was given refined steroids every few hours. His body broke out in huge welts. His veins began to collapse from the injections, and he could no longer raise his arms. He finally had to receive injections in his ankles.

One day, Ted learned that he was one of the first people to receive the steroids, and he realized he was being used as a human guinea pig. Ted became so angry and frustrated, he demanded to be sent home.

He tried three other doctors. None gave a single ray of hope. Ted developed ulcers and allergies. Then one day, Ted heard a radio program on nutrition. It recommended vitamins. He took some and felt slightly better. Gradually, Ted became aware that allopathy (orthodox medicine) was not the only therapy available. There were alternatives.

He investigated and sampled everything from acupuncture to chiropractic and homeopathy. Though Ted was far from cured, the alternative healing practitioners did something his doctors had failed to do. They advised him to stop drinking and smoking and to give up coffee and junk foods. Bit by bit, Ted improved. But he was still in pain and far from well.

At last, Ted learned about fasting. At age forty-one, he fasted for thirty-five days at a Hygienic institution in Texas. It was here that he experienced his first complete and lasting relief from pain.

Ted was so delighted that he became a dedicated Hygienist. He learned to accept complete responsibility for his own health. He also learned that his arthritis was the result of an underlying condition of toxemia caused by years of improper living and eating.

Since all medications are also toxic, the cortisone and

steroids his doctors had given him only worsened his tox-emia. Ted learned that Natural Hygiene still had no cure for arthritis. But unlike allopathy, it did offer a sure road back to health.

Once Ted had completely removed the cause of his toxemia, his arthritis began to lessen along with his ul-cers and allergies. In place of his former diet, high in fats, cholesterol, and refined carbohydrates, Ted now eats only fresh, raw fruits, vegetables, nuts, and seeds. He exercises vigorously for at least an hour each day.

Soon after his fast, Ted was well enough to return to college and graduate with a master's degree. Now at fifty-six, he enjoys glowing good health and an abun-dance of energy without a trace of stiffness or pain.

By turning to fasting and then adopting vegetarianism and exercise, Ted was merely rediscovering a natural health care system that was known and practiced in bi-blical times and even earlier. But the Hygienic move-ment did not begin officially until 1832 when Sylvester Graham, a young Presbyterian minister, assembled all the information then known on human physiology and health. He was soon joined by a number of prominent physicians such as Russell T. Trall and John H. Tilden, who recognized the fallacy of existing medical techniques. Tilden wrote *Toxemia Explained,* which is still a Hygienic classic. Hygienic doctors served in the Civil War and helped hundreds of wounded to recover more quickly.

After the Civil War, various branches of physical cul-ture and Nature Cure merged with the Hygienic move-ment. Numerous spas and fasting institutions were estab-lished, some licensed as medical schools. Hygienic books and periodicals flourished.

Toxemia then was caused more by poor sanitation and living conditions than by chemical pollution. Since the Roman era and earlier, people have managed to ruin their health by overeating, under-exercising, and leading dissipated lives.

After the 1870s, the medical profession became immersed in drugs, surgery, and seeking "cures." People found it more exciting to unbridle their appetites than to exert the discipline required to live in harmony with Nature. When they became sick, it was easier to go to a doctor and take a physic than to achieve genuine good health.

In the ensuing decades, when people believed that medical science had all the answers, Hygienic principles and knowledge were preserved and practiced by a relative handful of brilliant men and women. Every contemporary Hygienist acknowledges a debt to Dr. Herbert M. Shelton, the dean of Hygienic practitioners, who has successfully encouraged fasting in over 40,000 people and has set down the body of Hygienic knowledge in a series of self-help books.

In 1949, the American Natural Hygiene Society was founded to educate the public in Natural Hygiene. Local chapters were set up in most areas. Each year, a national convention is held where Hygienic techniques and advances are presented by such well known practitioners as Dr. Virginia Vetrano, Dr. William L. Esser and Dr. Alec Burton from Australia. Hygienists employ the title "doctor" in its original concept, meaning "teacher." Though most Hygienic practitioners today are chiropractors or licensed healers in alternative therapies, their main task is to teach the principles of healthful living.

The ranks of Hygiene are filled with people who were

once desperately ill and were told that medical science could do no more. By faithfully staying with Hygiene, many have made complete recoveries and have lived for decades after doctors pronounced them "incurable." Not all formerly sick Hygienists are totally restored to health but the majority are alive and functioning well. Many have already outlived their peers by ten or fifteen years.

Today's sweeping disenchantment with contemporary medicine began in the early 1960s when young people and adults by the tens of thousands turned to hatha yoga and sought tranquility in meditation. People rediscovered the pleasures of organic gardening and the joys of eating natural foods. A flood of "natural" health books appeared, promising fitness in a few minutes a day and instant health by eating "miracle" foods. Bookshops are filled with titles promising quick weight loss, rejuvenation, and total fitness by fragmented, unholistic methods that were designed to sell books rather than to provide any real, lasting benefit to readers.

Natural Hygiene Is A Health Care System Whose Time Has Come

If you're hoping to find such gimmick sections as "four foods that can help your gall bladder," or "the miracle herb that shrinks prostates" within these pages, you are reading the wrong book. Trying to break up gallstones with some "miracle" herb are obviously unholistic attempts to treat isolated parts of the body without considering the whole organism. Since both gallstones and benign prostate enlargement are caused by toxins, the holistic solution is to detoxify the entire organism by fasting, exercise, and by eliminating high risk foods.

People with such multiple ailments as arthritis, hypertension, impotence, and migraine headaches often find that they all disappear simultaneously when the cause of toxemia is removed. Take the case of Marge S., a California schoolteacher. At age forty, Marge was thirty pounds overweight and was suffering from frequent colds, chronic fatigue, periodic nausea, dental cavities, a weeping vagina, numbness in the extremities, inflammation of the inner ear, and constipation. Shortly afterwards, she experienced breast pains, and found a hard lump in one breast, ¾-inch in diameter. After examination by a Los Angeles medical clinic, she was advised to have the breast removed.

Instead, Marge conferred with a Hygienic practitioner, Dr. Gerald Benesh of San Marcos, California. Dr. Benesh recommended an extensive fast. During and after the fast, Dr. Benesh introduced Marge to the Hygienic way of life. Gradually, the lump began to shrink. It took a second major fast to finally eliminate Marge's toxemia and to reduce the lump to negligible size.

As her toxemia vanished, so did all of Marge's earlier complaints. Gradually, the pain and discomfort in her breast also disappeared.

Each year since 1960, Marge has taken short semi-annual fasts and has never strayed from the Hygienic lifestyle. Now slimmed down to fit into a size ten dress and feeling wonderfully fit and energetic, Marge has boundless energy for the active life of a teacher and housewife as well as for community involvement.

The literature is full of cases like Marge where Natural Hygiene has saved a woman from losing a breast. Can Natural Hygiene really reverse cancer?

When cancer actually exists, Dr. Herbert Shelton and most other Hygienic practioners believe it is not reversible. But almost all Hygienic practitioners have found that medical diagnosis, even biopsies, are not entirely reliable and a large number of cases are on record where tumors of the breast and other organs have shrunk or disappeared through Hygienic living. Practitioners tend to believe that these tumors were never really cancerous in the first place.

This possibility can be readily understood by the Hygienic explanation that cancer is the final stage in the progress of toxemia. Toxemia begins with enervation and progresses to toxicity, irritation, inflammation, ulceration, and fibrosis, to finally end in cancer. The first six stages are benign and reversible but cancer usually is not.

Every Hygienic practitioner has a file of case histories showing that when toxemia is eliminated, benign tumors begin to shrink. The speed with which they disappear depends on how advanced was the stage of toxemia. Tumors resulting from ulceration or fibrosis may require several extended fasts and a long period of Hygienic rehabilitation before they finally disappear. Sometimes a tumor will shrink only partially but cause no further harm as long as the person continues to live Hygienically.

Nonetheless, the number of cases of regression or remission of cancer by natural means is growing. Dr. Carl O. Simonton, a former U.S. Air Force physician and radiologist, reports very encouraging results in preventing re-occurrence of cancer by visualizing the immune system destroying cancerous growths as one meditates. The book *How I Conquered Cancer Naturally* by Eydie Mae, listed in the bibliography at the back of this book, is an inspiring case history of a woman who overcame breast cancer without drugs.

The experience of Hygienic practitioners is that some people who are diagnosed as having cancer actually have a benign growth. If you suspect cancer, it would be well to make very, *very,* sure that you really do have it before submitting to any medical treatment. A benign tumor or growth frequently responds to fasting by shrinking or disappearing altogether. Even without fasting, a non-cancerous growth may eventually shrink if the cause of toxemia is removed. The process may be speeeded up by using the visualization technique employed by Dr. Simonton, as described in Chapter X.

How To Get Started In Natural Hygiene

The best way to launch into Natural Hygiene is with a fast. Assuming you have read the cautions in Chapter V regarding who should *not* fast, you may begin with a short fast of one to four days, or even five days. Hygienists consider that five days is the maximum one should fast without the supervision of a Hygienic practitioner experienced in fasting.

If you are reasonably healthy, have only minor ailments, and are not more than 15 percent overweight, a short fast should give you a swift start on the road to permanent health. After the fast, go immediately onto a Hygienic diet as described in Chapter VIII and begin, very gradually, to work into a daily exercise program as outlined in Chapter IX. Be sure to study Chapters V, VIII, and IX in detail beforehand.

If you are more than 15 percent overweight and have more serious problems, provided you observe the cautions described in this book, you may also launch into Natural Hygiene in the same way. But you should also consider contacting a Hygienic practitioner as soon as possible for counselling on the advisability of a longer fast at a Hygienic institution.

Even if you cannot fast, or do not wish to, you can still get started into Natural Hygiene by changing over to a living food, all vegetarian diet and by commencing an exercise program. People have obtained great benefit from Natural Hygiene without ever having fasted. Or you might try the juice or mono-fruit diets described at the end of Chapter V. Results simply take a little longer.

Most people will probably prefer to make a gradual transition into the Hygienic diet, exercise program, and lifestyle. The important thing is to eliminate from your life, as quickly as possible, all of the sources of toxins described in Chapters II and III. If, while reading these chapters, you wondered when we were going to actually begin discussing Natural Hygiene, rest assured that these chapters on the causes of toxemia are required preparatory reading. Knowing how to avoid toxins in the first place is just as important as knowing how to purify a body after it is suffering from toxemia.

If you smoke or drink alcohol, or are hooked on caffeine drinks, elimination of these dangerous stimulants must take top priority. The Hygienic way to break these habits is through a fast and the method is covered in Chapter VI. A five-day fast should eliminate physical addiction to cigarettes without painful withdrawal symptoms, and you should undertake this essential step, on your own or at a Hygienic institution, at the very first opportunity.

Once you begin to eat, all animal-derived foods and refined carbohydrates should be eliminated from the diet. Hygienists do not eat *any* meat, fish, poultry, seafood, eggs, or dairy foods nor use salt, sauces, dressings, condiments, sugar, spices, or sweeteners. One of the benefits of a short initial fast is that all desire for these foodstuffs quickly disappears. Many people do cling to cooked vegetables and some whole grain cereals or bread for a week or two while completing the change to a diet composed entirely of living foods. Others find it takes as long as six weeks before their gastric juices and digestion become completely accustomed to a natural diet.

With your own initial detoxification accomplished by a fast, and with a transition to a proper diet and exercise under way, you are well on the way to attaining good health.

The chapters in this book are presented in the order in which you will probably prefer to progress step-by-step into Hygiene. Though daily exercise will relieve tension, it does not remove the cause. Chapter X describes how to program your mind to transform your personality from a stress-prone Type A individual into a relaxed Type B person. Various other chapters describe techniques for achieving greater sexual vigor, longer life, and successful retirement, thus rounding out the holistic aspect of Natural Hygiene.

The only specific treatment for any particular body part consists of special exercises to strengthen weakened muscles in the eyes and some yoga postures which stimulate the endocrine glands. Yoga, of course, is not Natural Hygiene. But hatha yoga—the branch of yoga which includes physical postures, meditation and vegetarianism—constitutes another highly successful holistic health care system. Many individual Hygienists use additional techniques borrowed from yoga.

Natural Hygiene does not guarantee results, nor does it claim to be a quick or painless way to get well or lose weight. People become sick only after years of abusing the body. A condition caused by ten years of wrong liv-

73

ing cannot always be reversed in ten days. Most people do experience benefits soon after starting into Natural Hygiene. But serious ailments often take longer to slip away. Always remember that unlike drugging, which violates the laws of biochemistry, Natural Hygiene simply aids Nature in restoring health.

Be prepared to stay with Natural Hygiene. Some people mistakenly believe that after a fast and a period of Hygienic eating and exercise, they can safely return to their former lifestyle. This never works. Back come the toxemia and the same ailments or disease. Every Hygienic institution has its regular customers who live Hygienically for several months, then return to their former toxic way of living. Within a year at most, they are right back where they began.

Natural Hygiene rejects all drugs, medications, medical treatment (except in case of injury), vitamin and food supplements, vaccines and inoculations, and blood transfusions. When all the body's biological needs are met—clean air, sunshine, pure water, exercise, raw vegetarian foods, rest, sleep, security, emotional tranquility, and freedom from stress—the living biological organism will heal itself.

All healing is done by the body. Cuts, burns, bruises, and broken bones heal themselves. When a doctor sets a broken bone, he does not heal it. Stitches merely hold torn tissue in place while the body itself does the healing. As Benjamin Franklin said: "God heals and the doctor takes the fee."

The purpose of Natural Hygiene is to set in motion the body's natural recuperative powers. This is done by excluding all possible toxins from reaching the organism on the one hand and by providing all possible biological necessities on the other hand. Through observing these simple rules, Natural Hygiene lets you live longer and enjoy optimum health throughout life; it helps people recover lost health; and it allows those who have never known good health to experience it. If you follow it faithfully, Natural Hygiene can remove all future fears and anxiety regarding your health.

There are other benefits. The average person who lives Hygienically can anticipate an active and productive life until well into the late eighties or even nineties. Your body will become slim, slender and attractive. Each morning you will wake up feeling fresh and bursting with energy and each night you will fall asleep like a healthy child. You need no longer spend tedious hours poring over cookbooks and hot stoves. There will be no more greasy dishes to wash. You need not worry about becoming old or senile or facing years of useless inactivity when you retire. Most Hygienists "retire" to a life of organic gardening or farming that is healthier and more active than their workday life.

Many Hygienists have cancelled their health insurance. Others report saving thousands every year on medical and dental bills. Soon after embracing Natural Hygiene, you may wish to hold a garage sale to dispose of such unnecessary appliances as your electric can opener, dishwasher, blender and mixer, electric frying pan, toaster, and electric blankets. The only powerdriven tool in our home is an electric drill. Many Hygienists cultivate large organic gardens without ever using powerdriven tools or equipment.

Hygienic Women Enjoy Painless Pregnancy

Due to the excessive risk of venereal disease, Hygienists

do not engage in promiscuous sex. Nor do they wish to create a life that might be ended by abortion.

Hygienic women almost invariably have children by natural birth, and breast feeding is taken for granted. Women whose whole bodies are healthy usually enjoy painless pregnancy and childbirth free of morning sickness. Menstrual troubles are also rarely a problem. Should a Hygienic woman in early pregnancy feel any sign of sickness or vomiting, she will go to bed early and fast for three or four days. This short period of abstinence almost always restores health. Longer fasts are not undertaken during pregnancy because of risk of injury to the baby.

Among children of non-Hygienic parents born in the U.S., by hospital delivery, one in fourteen was a birth defect. Although no statistics are available, birth defects among naturally born babies of Hygienic parents seem almost unknown. Hygienically raised, breast-fed babies also seem immune from Sudden Infant Death, the unexplained disease which suddenly kills apparently healthy infants. All of which seems to indicate that the only way to realize your birthright—a long and healthful life—is to start bucking the system as early in life as you can.

A Hygienist quickly learns body wisdom, that is, learning to "listen" to the body instead of rushing off to a doctor. In the unlikely event that a Hygienist feels a localized pain or feels under par, he will immediately rest and fast for three or four days. In most cases, health is quickly restored.

A New Design For Living

An article published recently in the *Wall Street Journal* stated that healthful ways of living and eating can achieve more than any medical breakthroughs or sophisticated equipment that is likely to be invented.

If you genuinely want to enjoy good health rather than just pay lip service to it, you must reshuffle your priorities, giving health top precedence. For without health, nothing else counts.

Changing over to a Hygienic lifestyle does not just mean cutting out everything that is harmful or fun. It means replacing foods and activities of dubious benefit with an entirely new design for healthful living. For every old habit you must drop, Natural Hygiene offers a healthful new habit to replace it.

Before becoming Hygienists, Robert J., a bank employee, and his wife Ellen, a dental technician, lived and ate conventionally, spent their evenings bowling, drinking beer, eating pizza, and on weekends they played golf.

Upon becoming Hygienists, the couple redesigned their entire lives, based on a whole set of entirely new habits. They did not consciously drop any of their former activities. But eating new, living foods left no room for conventional foods or pizza. Beer had no place in a new habit which consisted only of drinking water. Robert and Ellen's new habit of taking a brisk one-hour walk after finishing work left no time for lingering over coffee and cigarettes, which had previously filled this time slot.

They both soon became so fit that bowling seemed out of place. They took up ice skating, yoga, and square dancing instead. Through these activities, they made many new friends. The couple also joined a local outdoor club whose members went hiking, canoeing, or ski touring every Saturday. On Sundays, Robert and Ellen introduced another totally new habit—raising vegetables in their backyard. To learn more about gardening, they joined a local organic gardening club.

Neither Robert nor Ellen intentionally cut out any of their former activities. But their new lifestyle allowed no time for bowling, golf, pizza, or beer. Through their new activities, they tripled their total of friends and acquaintances. Their new friends did not smoke, drank sparingly, and seemed better educated and more interesting. After a few months, the couple found their new Hygienic lifestyle incomparably richer and superior in every way.

Rather than setting any drastic and unattainable goals, you will probably suceed better by making gradual changes and setting graduated goals you can live with. Almost everyone has found it easier to accept small but steady changes. If you decide to continue a bad habit in moderation, make sure it is for a very short time. There is no such thing as living wrongly in moderation. You cannot smoke or drink coffee in moderation and still be safe.

Most people manage to coast through their twenties and thirties without serious illness. Not until they are forty or so do they become sufficiently alarmed about their health to consider Natural Hygiene. At that age, most Americans are rather firmly established in their lifestyle. Changing firm habits of eating, drinking, and exercise requires motivation and determination.

Even after learning that their lifestyle is responsible for major hazards to their health, many people prefer to continue their lives unchanged. Dr. Michael E. DeBakey, a prominent Texas surgeon, noted at a recent symposium of the American Health Foundation that many of his patients, upon recovering from an illness, tended to resume their former lifestyle of indulgent eating, drinking, and smoking, ignoring the soaring blood pressure they could have kept normal.

Books and magazine articles such as *How to Live With Your Ulcer* or *How to Live With Arthritis* testify to our willingness to go on abusing the body rather than change our lifestyle and get better.

In Natural Hygiene, the mere acts of fasting, living on raw food, and exercising provide a tremendous boost to your self-discipline and morale. As you feel better and better, you will rapidly develop the character to say No to a gratification.

Most people are so programmed to seek stimulation and excitement that they attempt to find it in everything, including food. Hygienists, as well as yogis, aim for a life of calmness, peace, and tranquillity. This may sound like a sweeping, radical change but it can put living back into your life for the rest of your years.

The rewards of changing from health-wrecking habits to life-extending routines are so overwhelming that my wife and I have never considered any other alternative. After reading a Hygienic best-seller, Jack Dunn Trop's *You Don't Have To Be Sick*, in 1964, we were so impressed that within forty-eight hours, we had completely transformed our lives. We have never regretted the change and have seldom diverged from the Hygienic way of life since.

Natural Hygiene Gives You More Spare Time

You're probably wondering where you will get the time for exercising, growing sprouts, and other Hygienic activities. Once you give up such time-wasting habits as lingering over a cocktail or relaxing over a cigarette, when you no longer have to wait for hours in doctor and dentist offices or stay home sick, and when cooking and washing greasy dishes is no longer necessary, you should have more than enough time for Natural Hygiene. Many Hygienists also prefer more active recreations than watching TV. After becoming Hygienists, most people actually find they have *more* spare time than before.

Becoming a Hygienist doesn't mean you must become a social outcast. Dining out can be a gracious custom and in many restaurants today it is possible to order a salad and vegetable plate with a baked potato, all prepared to order without salt. David Stry, owner of Villa Vegetariana, a Hygienic fasting and vacation resort in Mexico, orders a grapefruit and an avocado salad when dining out. Many restaurants today have salad bars, and cafeterias always have a choice of vegetarian side dishes free of fat, cholesterol, and refined carbohydrates. Restaurant food may not be as beneficial as eating living foods at home. But you *can* dine out without incurring the high risks of fried food, eggs, steak, or seafoods.

Never try to advise other people to change their lifestyles. Let them ask, first, how you manage to stay so active and youthful. They may then decide to follow your example. If your spouse does not share your interest in Hygienic living, don't try to force your system on him or her. Let your partner see how fit and healthy you have become. Your spouse will probably soon become interested.

When both husband and wife opt for Hygiene, children can also be gradually steered towards Hygienic living. High risk foods and supermarket junk can be replaced by more wholesome fruits and vegetables, candy and sugar by figs and dates.

A wife or mother who becomes the only Hygienist in a family should experience no great problem in adhering to Hygienic routines. But where a husband goes Hygienic and his wife does not, the wife may experience disappointment upon finding that her spouse no longer appreciates her cooking. Hygienic husbands sometimes find they have to fix their own meals. Fortunately, fixing a Hygienic meal takes, at most, only a few minutes.

The Cost of Going Hygienic

Most Americans, we think, can obtain the benefits of Natural Hygiene immediately and without additional cost. The only possible extras might be the original outlay for a water distiller or for staying at a Hygienic institution should an extended fast be necessary. You might also need walking or jogging shoes and exercise attire. And it is possible you may wish to consult your doctors before fasting, exercising, or changing over to a Hygienic diet.

Offsetting these possible outlays are several distinct economies. Nuts and fruits are often not much cheaper than steak, but you will probably save a dollar or two weekly on food, especially if you previously used tobacco, alcohol, or coffee. Through replacing power-driven tools and garden machines with muscle-power, by making all short trips on foot or by bicycle instead of by car, and by spending literally nothing on medical care, the savings in a single year can more than offset most initial outlays for pure water or long fasts. Many Hygienists also save hundreds of dollars every year by raising their own organically grown fruits, vegetables, nuts, and seeds.

We also save substantial sums during vacations by not

eating in restaurants and by walking everywhere instead of taking sightseeing tours. Through becoming fit, we have also been able to take such wholesome vacations as canoe camping in the Minnesota wilderness, touring Europe by bicycle, backpacking in the Colorado Rockies, and ski touring in New England—all providing exhilarating exercise amid inspiring scenery at rockbottom cost. Taking the overview, we'd say that far from costing us anything, Natural Hygiene saves my wife and me *at the very least $1,000 per year!*

If You Wish To Join the American Natural Hygiene Society

A single book such as this can describe only the basic principles of Natural Hygiene. For a greater, in-depth study of Hygiene's many facets, the American Natural Hygiene Society has published a series of volumes, each dealing with each branch of Natural Hygiene. You might also like to join the Society and receive its monthly newsletter. The society may also be able to put you in touch with a local chapter through which you can meet other Hygienists in your area. The society's address is: American Natural Hygiene Society, 1920 Irving Park Road, Chicago, Ill. 60613.

5

Fasting

The Magic Way to Reverse Toxemia and Rebuild Health

Since her early twenties, Ethel T., had spent her weekends indulging in the "good life," drinking, smoking, and overeating. Finally, when she reached thirty-two, her toxemia became so acute that her immunological system broke down. Ethel was rushed to hospital with a fever and given antiobiotics. The fever soon subsided but Ethel's condition was diagnosed as a combination of diverticulosis and transverse colon colitis. She was placed on baby foods, belladonna, and phenolbarbitol for life. No doctor told her there was any alternative to a lifetime on drugs and baby foods. It was two years before Ethel learned about Natural Hygiene.

She was able to take off less than three weeks from work but she hastened to Dr. Esser's Health Ranch, a Hygienic institution in Florida. Here, she abruptly ceased taking medications and underwent a sixteen-day fast. Within a week, Ethel felt better than she had in years. By the time she broke the fast, many of her aches and pains had completely disappeared.

Dr. Esser, one of America's most experienced Hygienic practitioners, found Ethel still toxic and advised her to continue fasting. But Ethel had to return to work.

Ethel never again took baby food. She became a strict Hygienist, and her condition continued to slowly improve.

The following year, she obtained eight weeks of absence and returned to Dr. Esser's. This time, she fasted forty days. As her kidneys strained out the toxins, her urine turned a coffee color. The skin on her arms and legs peeled three times. On the thirty-fifth day, she threw up bile. She did not have a bowel movement for over five weeks. But Ethel knew she was getting better. Her pulse, which before her first fast occasionally raced up to 160, dropped to a slow, reliable 44 beats a minute.

By the fortieth day, her urine had cleared and her tongue was no longer yellow. Dr. Esser pronounced her toxin-free and Ethel broke the fast with a glass of orange juice. During the fast, Ethel's weight had dropped from 145 pounds to a mere 98. She had lost so much weight that there was no padding left in her behind and just sitting on her pelvic bones felt uncomfortable.

The second fast helped Ethel's body to make a complete recovery. Today, at age forty-nine Ethel is lissome, sun-tanned, and brimful of energy. She remembers with a laugh the doctor who told her that she would never be able to eat anything but baby food for the rest of her life. For fifteen years, she has eaten every fruit, vegetable, nut, and seed that she chose. Throughout that time, Ethel has faithfully followed the rules of Natural Hygiene and has not been ill for a single day.

Ethel's remarkable recovery, considered routine by Hygienic standards, occurred because fasting is the quickest and surest way to aid the body in restoring health.

Fasting itself does not cure anything. But within twenty-four hours of abstaining from food, profound biological changes occur in the body. Large amounts of blood and energy are relieved from the task of digestion. By fasting and resting, every system in the body is provided with a complete physiological rest. While the total organism spews out toxins through the lungs, mouth, and kidneys, every organ is able to rest and rejuvenate. During a Hygienic fast, the body takes in nothing but pure water, fresh air, and sunshine. As detoxification progresses, the body's recuperative powers become increasingly free to restore good health. Hygienists consider fasting the only natural way to get well when sick. As an old German proverb put it: "The illness that cannot be reversed by fasting, cannot be reversed at all."

In recent years, word has spread of dramatic health recoveries that have occurred during and after fasts. Some physicians have climbed on the bandwagon by offering medically supervised fasting for weight loss. But down through the years, when most people, including the medical profession, heaped scorn on natural ways to get well, the know-how and practive of fasting was preserved almost exclusively by Natural Hygienists.

Some physicians who conduct fasts are inexperienced Johnny-come-latelies by comparison to most Hygienic practitioners, and one day at a medically supervised fasting spa can cost as much as one week at the average

Hygienic institution. However, most people can safely fast for up to five days at home without spending a penny.

What Fasting Can Accomplish

Fasting invariably leads to rapid weight loss. Anyone who fasts off surplus weight and then switches permanently to the Hygienic lifestyle, will remain at optimum weight for the rest of his life—all without dieting of any kind.

But fasting—together with mental and physical rest—does nothing more than set the stage, providing the total organism with the ultimate opportunity for restoration of health. *Never forget that only the body can heal.* Fasting merely relieves the body of energy-consuming tasks, thereby allowing the organism to begin a process of self-purification. By ridding itself of toxins, the body eliminates its condition of toxemia, the underlying cause of most human ailments. Once the cause of disease is removed, the body's own recuperative powers are free to begin healing.

Hygienic records are filled with cases of people who, after fasting, experienced such improved vision that they were able to discard glasses worn for years. The files of Villa Vegetariana, a Hygienic institution in Mexico, are filled with such typical comments made by fasters as: "improved digestion and bowel action. . . clear eyes and complexion. . . reduced blood pressure. . . improved heart action. . . reduction of enlarged prostate. . . increased sexual vigor. . . improved sense of smell and taste. . . breathlessness has gone."

Russian doctors use short fasts to rid urban dwellers of toxic residues from automobile and industrial pollution, and they pioneered the use of longer fasts for restoring schizophrenics to normal health. Interestingly, the former schizophrenics must remain on a toxin-free diet for life. Otherwise, toxemia returns and the disease with it.

Staying on a Hygienic diet after a fast is relatively easy.

"While fasting, my palate was completely rejuvenated," a sixty-year-old lady told us after undergoing a seventeen-day fast at Villa Vegetariana. "My tongue became more sensitive to taste so that eating simple foods has become the greatest pleasure. I've lost all appetite for fats and sweets, and for animal-derived foods and processed junk. My palate turns naturally to fresh fruits, vegetables, nuts, and seeds."

Not all fasts are entirely free of discomfort, but side effects are trifling compared to those of surgery or drugs. You are not constantly hungry, as you are when on a diet, and most fasts *are* painless. After a few days, fasters experience a calm, restful feeling free of all tension and anxiety. Depression is replaced by euphoria, insomnia slips away and most people experience a wonderful feeling of deep relaxation. By the third or fourth day of a fast, most people feel better than they have in years.

How The Body Heals Itself During A Fast

Within a day after fasting commences, the body accelerates production of ketones—a product of the breakdown of fatty acids—into the bloodstream. As the ketones become more numerous, they suppress hunger. At the same time, ketones create a drugless "high." This is the same "high" during which, while undergoing long fasts, some people experience a spiritual renewal.

Once the organism begins expelling toxins, the organism starts to remedy chemical imbalances in both body and mind. The mind becomes wonderfully sharp and clear and seems perfectly in tune with nature. Worries and anxieties slip away. Blood pressure drops and you feel unbelievably relaxed.

Fasting provides a clear example of the interaction of mind and body. Though fasting is basically a physical process, it allows the organism to rebalance body chemistry and to remedy ailments normally considered purely psychological. Few psychologists consider exercise or diet as a factor in healing. Yet it is patently obvious that few people who enjoy dynamic physical health ever complain of mental health problems.

Because fasting affects your total well-being, Hygienists consider fasting both a science and an art. Within twenty-four hours of abstaining from food, the organs of elimination commence a thorough house cleaning. The kidneys free the lymph and blood of toxic excess and every cell in the body is gradually purified. Toxic wastes are excreted through every body opening. The breath becomes odorous and a white or yellow coating covers the tongue. Relieved of their normal toxic load, the kidneys are able to increase their output and the urine turns down.

During the first few days, the organism eliminates much surplus fluid. Weight loss is rapid. As autolysis proceeds, surplus fat tissues are broken down and the toxins accumulated in them released. As fasting progresses, reserves are broken down in reverse order of value. Fat cells go first, protein last. The fat in muscle cells is also removed, causing muscles to diminish in size. But, Hygienists claim, there is no atrophy or loss of integrity of muscle cells.

By the end of the second week, toxic excretion causes an acidosis crisis after which blood pH normalizes. While blood sugar levels may rise, cholesterol and blood pressure levels often drop dramatically. During a fourteen-day fast, diastolic blood pressure typically drops by ten points or more and cholesterol from, say, 225 to 175 mgs. per cent. The insulin level normalizes. And hormones such as serotonin and hearin are active as the body restores its chemistry. Cellular enzymes aid the liver to convert its stored glycogen (starch) to sugar and to distribute it to all body cells.

Critics of fasting—most of whom have never missed a meal in their lives—are fond of using the term "starvation" to describe fasting. These people fail to appreciate that the two terms are quite distinct. When eating ceases, fasting commences, and the body continues to fast as long as it lives on its stored reserves of fat. Toxins have a proclivity for fat, thus most toxins are eliminated as the body's fat tissues break down and as fats are drawn from muscle cells. When fat reserves are exhausted, almost all toxins have also been expelled from the organism. At this point, the urine becomes clear, the yellow-white coating disappears from the tongue, and the breath smells like a baby's.

These are the signs that toxemia has been eliminated and that the fast should be broken. At this stage, also, hunger reappears. It reappears because the stored reserves of fat are exhausted and the organism is about to begin to live off its vital reserves of protein. Once the body feeds off its protein, starvation commences. No Hygienic practitioner will fast a person to the point of starvation.

Although fasting is not recommended for wounds or

broken bones, wounds heal and bones mend while fasting. By observing thousands of fasts, Hygienic practitioners are convinced that the body's reserves are ample to maintain good health during a fast. Thus Hygienists disagree with physicians who give proteins, vitamins, and minerals to patients undergoing fasts. Hygienic practitioners report that virtually no deficiency disease has ever appeared during a supervised fast.

By giving patients protein, vitamins, and minerals, Hygienists claim that physicians are interrupting the body's purifying process and inhibiting elimination of toxins. Admittedly, most physicians who employ fasting do so only for weight loss and, theoretically, it would seem logical to prescribe supplements during a fast. From a Hygienic viewpoint, however, these supplements merely hinder the body's recovery. Most physician-supervised fasts do achieve weight loss, but elimination of toxemia is often far below Hygienic expectations.

Not all physicians fail to understand that fasting can purify the body as well as shed weight. Dr. Allan M. Cotts, author of *Fasting: The Ultimate Diet*, supports the Russian view that fasting allows the body to mobilize its defense mechanisms against many ills.

Nor are all physician-supervised fasting programs ultra-expensive. For example, Dr. Victor Vertes, Director of Medicine at Mount Sinai Hospital in Cleveland, Ohio, has successfully fasted over 800 people each of whom have lost one hundred pounds or more. The program recently cost only $7 per day on an out-patient basis and includes taking a protein powder five times daily. But the program is concerned only with weight loss.

Most doctors today are aware that fasting is medically acceptable for treating obesity. But many physicians still criticize fasting and consider it dangerous. Reasons given are that fasting may cause abnormal heart rhythm, low blood pressure, or acute gouty arthritis. Or that fasting may become compulsive. Or, more likely, that fasting is an unmedical way of reducing. In any case, every physician is likely to urge you to consult your doctor before beginning even a brief fast.

Whether or not you decide on prior medical approval before you fast, you are wasting your money if you go to a physician who does not approve of fasting. Before making up your mind, it may make better sense to read about who should *not* undertake a fast.

Who Should NOT Fast

In his book *Fasting: The Ultimate Diet* Dr. Allan M. Cotts first clears himself with the A.M.A., by stating that: "You should consult your doctor before beginning even a short fast, just as you would before beginning any diet." And Dr. Cotts continues: "Before starting a long fast, as before starting any long-term weight reducing diet, it is advisable to have a medical examination that includes a liver profile and an electrocardiogram."

After this disclaimer, Dr. Cotts states that he is often asked "Is fasting safe?" To which he replies: "It is certainly safe for almost everybody. Each person is adaptable to fasting in a different manner and degree. . . . Most people can fast safely for a month or longer."

One thing is certain. You should never fast without consulting a Hygienic practitioner or physician if you are emaciated or underweight, have a liver disease, or have had a recent heart attack. Nor if you have cancer—especially of the liver or pancreas—gout, cerebral disease, kidney disease, uncontrolled hypoglycemia, diabetes, undiagnosed tumors, any blood disease, T.B., and active pulmonary disease, anemia, bleeding ulcers, or any organic defect. This is not to say that fasting may not benefit some of these conditions. It simply implies that you should not fast without professional consultation and supervision.

Women should not fast while nursing a baby nor, except for an occasional day now and then, while pregnant. A short fast of up to four days will often relieve morning sickness during early pregnancy, but it should not be practiced regularly.

Babies, children, and teenagers should not fast without the approval of a Hygienic practitioner or physician. Healthy children may safely fast one day per week provided that on the other six days, their protein intake exceeds the required minimum by one sixth. Young people who do fast under supervision are advised to eat at least sixty to seventy grams of complete protein daily for several weeks afterwards.

If you have the slightest doubt as to whether it is safe for you to fast, you should ask your doctor if there is any medical reason why you should not fast. Phrased this way, he must give a Yes or No reply. You don't need to ask his opinion of fasting.

Remember that all medications are toxic and that you must cease taking medications during a Hygienic fast. The real question you may have to ask your doctor is whether he can take you off medication so that you can safely fast. If your doctor says No, consider going to another doctor who is more in tune with fasting. Or consult a Hygienic practitioner.

Provided you have not had a recent heart attack—or have heart disease with disproportionate thrombosis—

fasting is usually highly beneficial. As Dr. Shelton writes: "In the hundreds of cases of heart disease that I have watched through fasts of various lengths, all but a few have developed stronger and better hearts. Many of them, including so-called incurable ones, have become entirely normal."

Provided you have no fears or anxieties about it you will invariably find fasting safe and beneficial. A knowledge of the wisdom and logic behind fasting can dispel all worries concerning its safety. In any case, if you find it uncomfortable, or if you dislike it, you can always break the fast at any time. If you have any doubts about your ability to fast, first try a one day fast. You will then create the urge for longer fasts.

Always bear in mind that the medical profession approves of fasting only as a means of weight reduction. Hygienists employ fasting as the prudent course of action in case of disease. Whenever a Hygienist feels the onset of a cold, cough, chill, or minor ailment, he will go to bed and commence fasting. Usually, a short fast will prevent a minor ailment from becoming a major one. In case of an acute disease, such as pneumonia or pleurisy, Hygienists consider that fasting is the prudent course. Instead of losing strength while fasting, sick people usually gain strength during a fast. By the time a fast is broken, they are comparatively strong once more.

Any fast of more than five days should be made under experienced supervision, preferably at a Hygienic institution. If you decide to fast on your own for five days or less, try to select a quiet, restful place away from harassment or emotional stress. You must not allow friends, family, or neighbors, however well meaning, to dissuade you. Provided it is tranquil, your own home is the best and cheapest place. All that you need are pure water, fresh air and, if possible, a place to sunbathe.

Fasting itself is simple enough. You just do not eat anything! No fruit juice, chewing gum, herb teas, soft drinks, coffee, tea, or carob. You may drink as much pure water as you like. Smoking, of course, is strictly *tabu*.

Some fasting authorities say you should use enemas, saunas, or colonic irrigations. Some physicians suggest taking purgatives or laxatives just prior to the fast. None of these practices is Hygienic, and none is of the slightest benefit.

Instead, take a short daily bath in tepid water. Avoid a long, hot enervating soak. Brush your teeth without toothpaste twice daily and rinse out your mouth regularly, using only water. Keep the feet and body warm at all times. Short sunbaths are beneficial in any weather. But during summer, limit sunbathing to early morning and late afternoon hours. In cooler weather, when the sun is low, you may sunbathe for up to one hour each day. After the third week of a fast, most practitioners suggest reducing sunbathing to fifteen minutes per day. Under no circumstance become red or painfully sunburned.

You may fast in any season. If you need a fast, begin at once, regardless of the time of year. Some Hygienic institutions allow fasters to take short walks and light, easy exercise. For maximum benefit, however, you should rest as much as possible, preferably in bed or in a *chaise-lounge* outdoors in the shade.

Mental and emotional rest is vitally important. All stimulation should be avoided. Don't strain your eyes reading or watching TV, and try to avoid noise. Use the relaxation technique described in Chapter X, and forget all about anxiety and fear.

Fasting Is More Pleasant Than Feasting

About twelve hours after commencing a fast, a feeling of false hunger may appear. Genuine hunger pangs are impossible within this short time. What fasters experience is a gnawing in the stomach accompanied by a weak and empty feeling. After about 48 hours, the stomach realizes that it is not going to be fed, and the sensations subside.

Actually, feeling empty is far more pleasant than feeling stuffed full of food. The vacant feeling can be alleviated by sipping a cup of hot water. During a fast, your water supply should be unquestionably pure. Distilled water is safest. Otherwise, use clean rain water, soft spring water, or reliable bottled water. Mineralized spa water is not recommended by Hygienists. Avoid drinking very cold water. At some tropical Hygienic institutions, coconut water is used. Drink only when thirsty. It is not essential to flush out the system by drinking excessive amounts of water.

As the body begins to excrete toxins that may have taken years to accumulate, the tongue becomes coated, the mouth acquires a bad taste, the breath takes on an odor, and the urine turns dark. Accompanying these reactions may be such mildly uncomfortable symptoms as nausea, vomiting, headaches, sleeplessness, weakness, giddiness, skin eruptions, palpitation, or faintness. These symptoms are usually rare and of brief duration. They are not serious crises and seldom present any danger. They are simply reactions caused by biochemical changes occuring deep in the body. If they appear at all, they usually pass off by the fourth day. From then on the fast is usually comfortable and pleasant.

In rare cases, vomiting or diarrhea can occur as late as the fourth week of an extended fast. They are mild cleansing crises. Afterwards, the faster feels stronger and better. Should vomiting persist during a do-it-yourself fast and show no inclination to end, there may be danger of dehydration and the fast should be broken. If both vomiting and diarrhea occur together, risk of dehydration is greater. Should you vomit up the fruit or juice with which you break the fast, try changing to a different fruit or juice.

These minor side effects are all signs that the body is purifying itself. They are almost always transitory and seldom persist for more than a day or two. It is best not to give in unless vomiting or diarrhea are severe and prolonged. If a cold breaks out during a fast, it may be safely ignored.

Since you will not fast for more than five days without professional supervision, you may not experience the signs that show a fast should be ended. Even though a do-it-yourself fast seems to be progressing well, you should always break it by the end of the fifth day.

How A Fast Should Be Broken

The normal signals to break a fast appear when the tongue clears, a clean taste returns to the mouth, the breath smells sweet, and the urine is clear. At this time hunger will also return, and the body should be virtually cleansed of toxins.

A do-it-yourself fast should be broken immediately if hunger persists beyond the fourth day, if you feel intestinal spasms or cardiac asthma, if you have a persistent high pulse rate, or if you experience prolonged weakness, dizziness, headaches, vomiting, and diarrhea.

While short fasts of up to five days or so are clearly beneficial, results are not nearly as spectacular as if you permit the fast to run its full undisturbed course. Many people must break a fast because of lack of time to complete it. A fast prematurely interrupted is better than no fast at all. But like Ethel T., you should plan to return later and allow your fast to run its natural course. Some people fast for sixty days or more before all surplus weight and toxemia have been eliminated.

A fast of not longer than fourteen days duration should be broken with a full glass of freshly squeezed fruit or vegetable juice. Follow this with a full glass of the same juice every two hours. It is not mandatory to drink this much unless you need it. Stay with fruit and vegetable juices for forty-eight hours. On the third day, eat two oranges for breakfast, two for lunch, and three for dinner. On the fourth day, you can begin eating fruits and vegetables. On the fifth day, you can commence a full Hygienic diet but increase the amount of food gradually. By the seventh day, you should be eating normal-sized Hygienic meals.

No activity should be scheduled for several days after breaking an extended fast. Activity can be resumed much sooner after a fast of five days or less.

After breaking a fast, stay religiously with the Hygienic diet and do not overeat. Most people experience an increased appetite after breaking a fast and tend to gorge. By eating only fruits, vegetables, nuts, and seeds, it is almost impossible to become overweight. But try not to overeat before your normal appetite returns.

Critics of physician-supervised fasts complain that after breaking the fast, patients begin to eat heavily and are soon overweight again. On a Hygienic diet and exercise routine, this is next to impossible.

Soon after a fast is broken such chronic complaints as sinus trouble or headaches frequently disappear for good. The eyes sparkle and their whites become clear. Graying and balding usually ceases and the hair takes on a healthy luster. Gradually your weight returns to its ideal level and remains there as long as you continue to eat and live Hygienically.

The Wonderful Benefits Of A Short Twenty-Four Hour Fast

Paul Bragg, who lived to be ninety-five and who wrote The Miracle of Fasting at age eighty-five recommended that everyone should fast for one day each week.

A short weekly fast provides a welcome rest for the entire body. The stomach becomes accustomed to feeling empty so that during longer fasts, side effects are seldom, if ever, experienced.

Besides cutting 15 percent from your food bill, a one-day weekly fast will boost your will power and eliminate any possibility of a chronic digestive condition.

Besides fasting once a week, some Hygienists also fast for two to three days each month or for ten days every six months. Paul Bragg recommended fasting for seven to ten days at a time on two, three, or even four occasions annually to maintain the organism in top condition.

For a one-day fast, you can continue your normal activities. Instead of jogging, we practice less strenuous hatha yoga postures on fast days. Some fat-farm directors encourage exercise to speed weight loss while fasting.

But Hygienists consider that strenuous exercise only hinders the expulsion of toxins during a longer fast.

How Fasting Can Reverse Arthritis

A small but growing number of M.D.s who specialize in arthritis are finding that the disease can be reversed by eliminating certain foods. The problem foods include beef and other meats; milk, cheese, and high-fat dairy foods; white bread and sugar; and, occasionally, such cereals as wheat, corn, and oats. None of these, of course, is eaten by Hygienists. An allergy to one or other of these foods is considered by many diet-oriented specialists as the cause of arthritis.

Not every arthritis sufferer is allergic to the same foods. To find out specifically which foods cause arthritis, the specialists have borrowed a traditional Hygienic technique. They place their patients on a five-day fast. After a few days without food, almost all patients report complete relief from arthritis pains. Patients then break the fast by eating only a single food, such as bread. If they remain free of pain, they are assumed non-allergic to bread. Next, another food is added, such as corn. Step by step, other foods are added. The food that precipitates a return of arthritic pain is considered a culprit and is eliminated from the diet.

Writing in the *Journal of Applied Nutrition,* Dr. Robert Bingham of the National Arthritis Medical Clinic in Desert Hot Springs, California, says: "Good diet and the elimination of bad foods can end the suffering of approximately 70 percent of arthritis victims."

Since nothing in the Hygienic diet appears to cause arthritis, you can streamline this cumbersome medical process by fasting for five days and then staying permanently with the Hygienic diet and lifestyle. A five-day do-it-yourself fast should end most arthritic pains for good. It will take longer, of course, for the joints to become supple and the swelling to disappear. Permanently damaged or twisted joints may never return to normal. But thousands of arthritics *have* made complete recoveries through Natural Hygiene, often in just a few weeks.

The Amazing Juice Fast

Comedian Dick Gregory recently ran from Chicago to Washington D.C., covering as much as forty miles per day, while living exclusively on fruit and vegetable juices. Earlier, Dick had lived on juices for over a year while protesting the Vietnam War. During this time, he completely eliminated all stimulants, brought his weight down from 300 to 140 pounds, and became an accomplished distance runner.

If for some reason you simply cannot fast, you can attain a good many of the benefits of fasting by going on a juice "fast." By Hygienic standards, a juice "fast" is no fast at all. More properly, it should be called a "diet." Yet it does ease the burden of digestion, and it also provides the organism with a physiological rest comparable, though not equal to, that experienced during a genuine fast.

If you decide to try a juce fast, you may drink as much juice as you need to feel comfortable. Use only freshly-squeezed juices, and plan to use at least as much vegetable as fruit juices. Do not mix fruit and vegetable juices. After drinking a fruit juice, wait a full hour before taking a vegetable juice, and vice versa.

You can count on losing three to five pounds a week during a juice fast. Since elimination of toxins is a slower process, there is no need for bed rest. You can continue your daily activities.

Ascertain your ideal weight and end the juice fast before or when your weight drops to this level. Do not stay on a juice diet indefinitely because it too lacks protein. Should you experience prolonged diarrhea or other discomfort, common sense suggests switching to a genuine fast for a day or two till health is restored.

Don't expect the dramatic results of a Hygienic fast. But a juice diet has helped thousands of people to regain normal weight and to reverse their less severe problems. The process simply takes longer.

The Benefits of Fasting While You Continue To Eat

George F., had suffered for years from impotency and an enlarged prostate. At sixty-eight, he was flabby, paunchy, partially deaf, and wore thick glasses. He walked with a pronounced stoop, his sinuses dripped continually, and he wheezed with bronchial asthma. George F., had been taking several different medications for over seven years. Yet he had felt no improvement and, in fact, was slowly becoming worse.

One day, George read a book that described how health could be restored by eating nothing but a single fruit. The recommended fruits were papaya, grapes, or watermelon. The book told how the diet had been successfully used at several health spas in Europe and Mexico to restore the health of people who preferred not to fast.

The markets were filled with watermelons in the small Colorado town where George lived. So he bought a supply and gave the diet a try. His doctor had said it wouldn't hurt to drop his medications for a month or two. According to the book, George was allowed to eat all the fruit he wanted provided it consisted entirely of one type of fruit.

For three weeks, George ate nothing but watermelons. He drank no beverages, took no salt or condiments, and no medication. He was allowed to drink all the pure water he required. But the watermelon supplied most of his fluid requirements. He munched watermelon as often as eight times a day. George never felt hungry. But in three weeks, he had lost twelve pounds, and he felt a whole lot better.

Following the book's instructions, he began to take a brisk walk every day. Each day, he walked farther and faster. By the sixth week, George noticed that his glasses seemed too strong. His wheezing had stopped and so had his sinus drip. He no longer felt any prostate discomfort and seldom had to get up in the night. His doctor was amazed at the improvement. George stayed on the mono-fruit diet for another two weeks. By then, his hearing had begun to improve and for the first time in eight years, he became sexually active.

The book directed George to stay on a diet of natural vegetarian foods for the rest of his life. That was several years ago. Now, lean and upright, George swings along with a relaxed stride and except for wearing weaker glasses, is almost totally recovered.

Over the years, thousands of people have benefited from the mono-fruit diet. It is still a popular therapy at "nature cure" spas in Europe and elsewhere. By eating only a single fruit, the task of digestion is reduced to its barest simplicity. Except that it provides something solid instead of mere liquid, it does not differ appreciably from the all-juice diet.

As George discovered, a mono-fruit diet can achieve

many of the benefits of a Hygienic fast. Like the juice diet, results simply take longer. The same cautions apply as with a juice diet. A mono-fruit diet should not be continued indefinitely.

Watery, pulpy fruits such as melons, papaya, or grapes are most suitable. In lieu of these, apples or pears might be used.

Zen Buddhists report similar purifying effects after living temporarily on a diet of nothing but cooked, unrefined rice. In fact, a rice diet has been successfully used by some weight loss clinics. For that matter, a diet of nothign but boiled potatoes over a period of, say, three to four weeks would probably prove far more beneficial than the standard American diet.

A REMINDER: that no one should ever fast for more than five days without experienced professional supervision. Study this chapter in detail before attempting any do-it-yourself fast and carefully read the section "Who Should NOT Fast." The same cautions outlined in "Who Should NOT Fast" are equally applicable to anyone contemplating a fruit juice or mono-fruit diet.

Let's Start Detoxifying

The Painless Way to Phase Out Cigarettes, Alcohol or Coffee

Going on a fast to stop smoking seems to make about as much sense as putting on a hat if your feet get cold. But since one fifth of our blood is circulating through the head at any one time, putting on a woolen hat does help your blood to warm up. In a few minutes, the extra warmth reaches the feet. Likewise, few smokers have any urge to light a cigarette, or to have an alcoholic drink or a cup of coffee, on an empty stomach.

By going on a fast, the problem of how to stop smoking or drinking becomes a new problem: how to keep from eating. It's a whole lot easier to stop eating for a few days than to stop smoking or drinking alcohol or coffee.

Many nutritionists believe that inadequate nutrition is the basic reason why people continue to smoke or drink.

During a fast, the entire organism excretes accumulations of nicotine or caffeine more rapidly than by any other method. Withdrawal symptoms are minimal. When you fast, you quickly sense that stimulants will only destroy the wonderful feeling of lightness and freedom that comes with not eating. Your taste buds are totally transformed during a fast. Even after you begin to eat again, cigarettes, snuff, alcohol, or coffee will no longer taste good.

The length of time you need to fast to stop smoking or drinking is, usually, only five days. Writer Lorraine Dusky, reporting on a five-day fast at Villa Vegetariana in *Town & Country Magazine,* said that she hadn't had a cigarette, nor the least desire for one, since beginning the fast. When she tried lighting up her favorite menthol cigarette after breaking the fast, it tasted like poison.

Normally, you need not go to a Hygienic institution for a fast to eliminate stimulants. Since the required fast should not exceed five days, it can be carried out at home without cost. Fred M., tells how he was a two-pack-a-day smoker for twenty years. After fasting at home for only five days, all desire for cigarettes had disappeared. That was seven years ago, and he has not smoked since.

One thing is essential. After breaking the fast, you must stay with a strict program of Hygienic eating and living. One toxin invariably leads to another. If you begin eating animal-derived foods or refined carbohydrates, the body will soon feel sluggish and the desire for stimulants may return.

Experience shows that those who drink coffee and smoke cigarettes are also more likely to become regular users of alcohol. The Hygienic solution is to eliminate all stimulants simultaneously and to detoxify the body at the same time. For most addicts, a fast will accomplish more in five days than most anti-smoking or anti-drinking systems do in five months. For those who stay with Natural Hygiene, the drop-out rate is virtually zero.

During the times we have spent at Natural Hygiene conventions, not once have we seen a Hygienist light up a cigarette or drink coffee or alcohol. Not a trace of cigarette smoke marred the lecture halls or eating areas.

Students of hatha yoga also report that they frequently find it almost impossible to equate taking stimulants with the wonderful feeling of lightness and peace that yoga brings. Merely by becoming vegetarian and practicing yoga deep breathing, all urge to smoke or to drink stimulants slips away. Fasting, followed by Hygienic diet and exercise, is just that much quicker and more certain.

Since almost everyone who smokes or drinks stimulants is already sick to some extent, fasting to eliminate stimulants does not differ from fasting to recover from any other form of ill health. The fast should be undertaken exactly as described in Chapter V. Since stimulants are so hazardous to your health, your doctor will probably cooperate fully by granting you medical permission, if you need it, before undertaking the fast.

Because so many smokers and drinkers, including coffee drinkers, are so heavily afflicted with toxemia, a five-day fast will not normally be sufficient to completely detoxify the organism. If you can spare the time, it is always advisable to fast until the body is completely purified. This will mean fasting at a Hygienic institution. Failing this, you should embark on a do-it-yourself fast of no more than five full days in order to eliminate stimulants as rapidly as possible. Partial detoxification will occur during this time and any detoxification is preferable to no detoxification at all. By living and eating Hygienically after the fast, detoxification will also continue, albeit at a more gradual pace.

If you have already tried unsuccessfully to quit smoking or drinking, you will probably find it hard to believe that simply by fasting, all urge to smoke or drink will disappear. Yet thousands of Hygienists and others have quit this way and for those who remain staunch Hygienists afterwards, the number of backsliders has been negligible.

How Fasting Destroys All Craving for Cigarettes, Alcohol and Coffee

During a fast, the body undergoes such powerful biochemical changes that alcohol and cigarettes become repugnant to the taste. Going without food for several days invariably produces such a euphoria that the usual withdrawal symptoms are not experienced at all. Life changes so completely after a few days of fasting that smoking or drinking becomes unimportant.

As you quit smoking, your metabolic rate will probably slow. To compensate, most people tend to overeat and add weight. After breaking the fast, you may also find yourself eating more fruits, vegetables, nuts, and seeds. If so, don't worry! Regardless how much you eat, it is difficult to add weight on a high fiber diet. Go ahead and eat all you want for a while. Cigarettes are so life-threatening that almost any minor indulgence is preferable to smoking.

The same observation applies to anyone with a drinking problem. David Reuben, M.D., reports in his book *The Save Your Life Diet* that after switching to a high fiber diet, many drinkers find that within a month their desire for alcohol has almost disappeared.

After breaking the stimulant habit, you may find that instead of responding to a situation of anxiety, stress, or boredom with a cigarette, cocktail, or cup of coffee, you eat compulsively instead. Don't worry about this either. It's almost impossible to seriously harm the body by overeating on Hygienic foods.

Once you are safely over the stimulant addiction, you can easily remedy compulsive eating by using the relaxation techniques described in Chapter X. Instead of responding to anxiety or monotony by eating, use muscular relaxation and deep breathing.

Start A New Habit—Non-Smoking

Consider your transformation not as simply cutting out smoking but as beginning a *new* habit of non-smoking. Try to select a time for your fast when you are free of anxieties and emotional stress. If you are not able to go on a fast almost immediately, you may be able to quit cold turkey right away. It is not as easy as using a fast but almost one person in two is able to stop smoking using only the Sudden Stop method.

If you try it, start each day with a glass of freshly-pressed citrus or pineapple juice. Replace all customary cups of coffee, tea, chocolate, cola drinks, or alcohol with fresh fruit or vegetable juice. Whenever you feel the urge to smoke, take a dozen deep breaths instead. Each evening, go for a long, brisk walk. Work hard at some physically tiring task. Exercise can substitute for nicotine by speeding up heart action, which smoking also does. But exercise does it safely.

Remove all ashtrays and matches from the house and

all cigarettes but one. (Keep on hand a single cigarette of the brand you hate most just to provide the assurance of knowing that you can smoke it if you want to.) Tell all your friends you are giving up smoking. Make a list of the reasons why you want to quit smoking and read them every time you feel like lighting up. Quit smoking for only one day at a time. The following day, try for another day of non-smoking. The first two days are most difficult. Lay in a supply of fruits, dates, figs, even chewing gum or fruit cake if you like. If you can achieve five smoke-free days, you've made it.

Even though you are aiming only to stop smoking, you will also have replaced the alcohol and coffee you normally drink with juices. At the end of the week, you should have broken dependence on *all* stimulants.

Don't be afraid to exercise while becoming a non-smoker. Walk, ride a bicycle, or paddle a canoe amid beautiful, restful scenes. The wonderful feeling of well-being that results will boost morale.

How To Start Feeling Better Almost Immediately

You should make quitting stimulants the number one priority of your life. If you have been a smoker, your risk of experiencing a heart attack is reduced *immediately,* even if you have already had a heart attack or angina. Symptoms of chronic bronchitis and emphysema soon begin to fade and progress of these diseases is retarded. Coughing and wheezing soon stop while taste and smell are immeasurably improved. After three or four days, you will experience a noticeable increase in energy and you will sleep through the night.

Twelve months after you stop smoking, risk of lung cancer begins to decrease until, after being a non-smoker for ten years, your risk has dropped almost to that of non-smokers.

Stimulants exert a grim synergistic effect. If you both smoke *and* drink alcohol, the combined risk makes you many times more prone to disease. A person who both smokes and drinks heavily runs five times the risk of contracting oral cancer as a person who does only one of these things.

If you smoke and also have a high fat diet, you are running nine times the risk of contracting a degenerative disease than if you merely smoked and had a low fat diet. If you smoke and don't exercise, your risk of ill health is 33 percent higher than if you smoked and exercised. If you smoke, drink alcohol and coffee, eat a high fat diet, and don't exercise, you are running a tremendous risk. Yet this profile fits almost one American in two. Just about all Americans, including children, are hooked on caffeine. Several studies have shown that drinking beverages containing caffeine increases the risk of heart disease and diabetes and has been linked with several types of cancer.

If you find it difficult to give up tea, coffee, chocolate, cocoa, or cola drinks, use fresh fruit or vegetable juice instead. Or try using carob or a herb tea like linden or peppermint. These non-stimulant drinks are sold in health-food stores. Make sure the carob is sugar-free.

Studies show that nine out of every ten smokers woud quit if there was an easy way out. Well, there is. It is called Natural Hygiene! The benefits of becoming a non-addict are so overwhelming that you should not hesitate to go on a stimulant-ending fast at the very first opportunity.

A REMINDER: that no one should ever fast for more than five days without experienced, professional supervision. Study Chapter V in detail before attempting any do-it-yourself fast and carefully read the section "Who Should NOT Fast."

7

The Natural Hygiene Way to Become Slim, Slender and Attractive

On January 1, 1975, Joan R., weighed a hefty 260 pounds and looked ten years older than her forty-six years. Joan had not always been overweight, but after a hassling divorce in 1968, she'd had to take a job on a newspaper in Chicago. The frantic pace of newspaper work proved so demanding that eating obsessively seemed to provide the only relief. Whenever she felt unhappy or unloved, she would head for the refrigerator. For two years, she tried diet after diet but always ended up by adding weight instead of losing it. Finally her brother, a natural Hygienist, mentioned fasting.

In mid-January 1975, Joan took off four weeks from her job and fasted for twenty-five days at Vegetariana, the Hygienic institution in Mexico. She lost thirty-six pounds. While at Villa Vegetariana, she learned to live and eat Hygienically. Over the next six months, she lost an average of almost two pounds a week, despite eating all the fruits and vegetables that she desired.

By now, Joan realized that to keep her health, she'd have to switch to a slower paced occupation. In August, she returned to Villa Vegetariana and fasted for another sixteen days. She lost another twenty pounds. Back in Texas, she found a low-keyed job clerking in a healthfood store. She went on eating Hygienically and continued to lose a little over a pound each week.

On December 31, 1975, Joan weighed a trim 136 pounds, felt better than she had in years, and looked about thirty-eight. Altogether during 1975, she lost a total of 124 pounds; 56 pounds while fasting, at an average weight loss of 1.36 pounds per day; and 68 pounds while eating Hygienically, at an average rate of 1.5 pounds per week.

For her medium frame and 5'8" height, her new 136-pound weight looked just right. And it must have. Because early in 1976, she met and married a Hygienist only two years her senior. The pounds had melted away without leaving any flabbiness or sagging.

At any one time, approximately twenty million Americans as on a weight-reducing diet. Only one in four actually ever loses weight, and many of these soon put it back on. Joan succeeded because she elected fasting—the swiftest, most dramatic way to lose weight—and because she followed it by living Hygienically, the most successful holistic weight control system in existence.

The Longer The Waistline, The Shorter The Life

Joan was also lucky in being able to regain her normal weight before her obesity caused a serious illness. Since toxins have a proclivity for fat, an obese person rapidly builds up a dangerous level of toxemia. American men who are only 10 percent overweight increase their chance of premature death by 20 percent. On balance, men 10 percent and more overweight run an inceased risk of dying from heart attack by 142 percent (women by 175 percent); from stroke by 149 percent (women 162 percent); from liver or gallbladder cancer by 168 percent (women 211 percent); and from diabetes by 383 percent (women 372 percent). They also increase their risk of a hernia by 154 percent (women 141 percent); of chronic nephritis by 191 percent (women 212 percent; and of cirrhosis of the liver by 249 percent (women 147 percent).

In its official publication, *The Challenge of Cancer,* the National Cancer Institute recently stated: "There is statistical evidence from several insurance companies that overweight people have a greater tendency for developing cancer."

Shedding weight is big business. Medically supervised fat farms charge up to $1,000 a week, and you may still lose only five to ten pounds. Fad diets become the rage for a few months till people learn they cannot stay with them.

Low carbohydrate diets, no-aging diets, grapefruit diets, 1,000-calorie diets, starvation diets, high fat diets—all produce some weight loss at first. But they are all nutritionally unsound and based on fallacious principles of body physiology and psychological weight control. Over half the diets are dangerously high in protein, fats and cholesterol, and they significantly increase the risk of eventually incurring a degenerative disease.

Most people find these diets so monotonous that they

cannot live with them. All the diets concentrate on losing weight instead of in lowering the Appetite Control Center (ACC). To lose weight and to *keep* it off requires a holistic approach that includes exercise, sound nutrition and a diet low in fats, protein, and refined carbohydrates. Fasting, followed by Hygienic living, meets all these requirements.

Fasting, also, is probably the only weight loss method through which subtle endocrine changes occur which accelerate the metabolic rate and slow down conversion of glucose into fat—and which persists long after the fast.

A recent study at Rockefeller University revealed that fat people have up to three times more fat cells than people or normal weight. The preponderance of adipose cells is the result of overeating in childhood. Compared to children of normal parents, only 10 percent of whom are overweight, in families where one parent is overweight, 50 percent of the children are overweight. When two parents are overweight, 80 percent of the offspring are overweight. Researchers consider that obesity is not inherited but is learned from obese parents who overeat of the same fatty diet fed to the children.

Overeating fatty foods during childhood creates a surplus of fat cells whose demands for food stimulate the ACC to provoke hunger pangs. The extra fat cells are also quite difficult to get rid of. Something more than mere weight loss is required for lasting weight control.

Whether seeds of overweight were sown in childhood or acquired later, our weight is actually controlled by our ACC. Regardless how much we eat or exercise, the ACC normally maintains our weight within a pound or two of its current setting. It also controls our hunger.

The actual weight level maintained by the ACC is

strongly influenced by the proportion of fat cells. It is also affected by levels of physical activity, emotion, and metabolism. Feeling unhappy or unloved, anxious or tense, can drive up the ACC level. When this happens, the ACC sends out hunger signals which trigger compulsive or obsessive eating. Fat cells also become hungry and send messages to the ACC for more food, especially fatty food.

Exercise, by contrast, benefits the whole body and causes the ACC level to drop. Lasting weight loss will occur only if the ACC level is permanently adjusted downwards. Only through a holistic program of natural living and eating, with abundant exercise, will the ACC adjust itself to a lower level.

By fasting, you can lose twelve to eighteen pounds in a mere ten days without feeling hungry. By eating only living vegetarian foods after the fast, you can eat all you want without ever having to count calories. Week by week, you will gradually lose weight until your ACC level adjust to maintain your ideal weight. In losing weight, it is especially important to adopt the complete Hygienic lifestyle, not merely to eat Hygienically. Regular daily exercise is an essential factor in changing the body's metabolic process and in permanently lowering the ACC level. As soon as possible, you should also attain emotional tranquillity and a relaxed attitude through practicing the techniques in Chapter X.

How To Lose At Least A Pound A Day By Fasting

Fasting for weight loss is essentially the same as fasting for any other reason. You take absolutely no food, beverages, stimulants, or anything else except all the pure water you need. Complete instructions for carrying out a do-it-yourself fast are given in Chapter V. Be sure to study this chapter in detail, especially the section entitled "Who Should NOT Fast."

Ideally, a fast for weight loss should also be allowed to run its full natural course until the whole body is completely purified and all accumulated toxins eliminated. For a person thirty pounds overweight, such a fast might last a month. More than the required thirty pounds might be lost before all toxemia is expelled. After the fast is broken, the ACC would gradually increase weight to the ideal level. Such an extended fast should be undertaken only when supervised by a Hygienic practitioner experienced in fasting.

While fasting people for weight loss, physicians often encourage the faster to exercise and even to continue working. Physicians usually prescribe vitamins, minerals, and powdered proteins while fasting. When weight loss is the main reason for fasting, some Hygienic practitioners also permit fasters to take walks or light exercise.

Lacking the necessary time or funds to fast under supervision, you may, alternatively, undertake a five-day fast every second week. This, of course, assumes you have your doctor's permission to fast or that you are convinced you do not need it. For example, you can safely fast from Tuesday night until Monday morning, breaking the fast with fruit juice on Monday morning and taking nothing but fruit juice all day Monday. Then on Tuesday, you can begin eating Hygienically, on a moderate scale. By Wednesday, you can resume full-scale Hygienic eating and continue for a full week until, by the following Tuesday night, you are ready for another five-day fast.

This program is not nearly as ideal as a longer, unbroken fast. Yet it *is* the next best thing, and it *will* produce results. Using this alternate eating-fasting program, most overweight people can expect to lose about fourteen pounds per month. Be sure never to fast more than five days at a time without qualified supervision and never for more than ten days in any four week period. Avocadoes should be excluded from the diet and you should substitute sprouted beans and grains, and cooked soybeans for nuts and seeds until your weight reaches normal levels.

While fasting, you will lose weight rapidly during the first two to three days. Typically, you may lose five pounds the first day and three more the second day. Such large losses during the first few days are due to the body eliminating large amounts of water and also feces, which are not replaced. After a few days, weight loss drops to about one pound per day. After fasting thirty days, an overweight person may easily shed up to 20 percent of body weight. Thereafter, weight loss gradually decreases. During the final days of an extended fast, the loss may be as little as one fourth pound per day.

If you are using the do-it-yourself method just described, you should ascertain your ideal weight in advance. Usually, your best weight is one to two pounds below the average weight published in height-weight tables. Stop all fasting when you have reached this level.

Except that a short five-day fast can be broken more rapidly than a longer fast, weight-loss fasts are broken in the same way as any other fast. Consult Chapter V for details.

How To Tell If You Are Overweight

People with large frames and big bones can weigh fifteen pounds or more than a lightly built person of the same height and still not be overweight. If you are not certain whether you actually are overweight, try this simple pinch test.

Pinch a fold of your flesh by lifting it free of the underlying tissue and measure the thickness of the pinched fold. Make pinch tests at the waist, stomach, calf, buttocks, and under the upper arm. The pinched fold should not be more than .5-1 inch thick. If over an inch, you are carrying too much fat for your skeletal frame. If under half an inch, you are underweight.

If you are too fat and your weight is higher than your best weight based on height-weight tables, you are probably overweight. A supervised fast is recommended or, failing that, a combination of five-day fasts alternated by Hygienic eating and exercise. If you are too fat but not overweight, you are simply too flabby. The remedy here is to convert the fat into muscle through exercise. You should eat Hygienically but no fasting is required—at least, not for weight loss. A combination of walking or jogging plus upper-body calisthenics—arm and trunk exercises—are ideal for converting fat into muscle uniformly all over the body.

If you are both under-fat and underweight, you should also begin to eat Hygienically and to exercise. You should increase the amount of avocadoes in your diet and you should be sure to eat your daily allocation of nuts and seeds. However, a skinny, emaciated figure may be due to impaired digestion and food assimilation caused by toxemia. Curiously, a supervised fast can often eliminate the toxemia so that when eating recommences, weight gain is quite rapid. A fast for gaining weight should be undertaken only at a Hygienic institution.

When eating resumes, you can increase the amount of avocadoes, nuts, and seeds in the diet.

Overweight people often blame their eating habits on an over-active thyroid gland. Usually, this is putting the cart before the horse. What often happens is that, as a result of overeating, thyroid activity becomes impaired. After normal weight is regained, the thyroid gland usually resumes normal activity.

How To Walk Your Pounds Away

One pound of body fat contains 3,500 calories. To maintain this amount of fat consumes another 15 calories per pound of body weight per day, assuming moderate activity. Thus a 160 pound man requires 2,400 calories per day to maintain normal weight. (It is interesting to note that though these figures are considered entirely dependable in America, the daily intake of older Abkasians and Vilcabambans—who are more active than most Americans—is only 50-75 percent of these amounts.)

On this basis, there are two ways to get rid of fat. First, if you burn up 100 calories a day through exercise, you will lose one pound in thirty-five days. Second, if you eat 100 fewer calories per day, in thirty-five days you will also eliminate one pound of fat.

An hour of rowing burns up 675 calories, while an hour of jogging or swimming the crawl consumes 600 calories. Through burning 600 additional calories a day in exercise, you will lose a pound in slightly less than six days. That means ten pounds in two months.

Brisk walking at 3.5 m.p.h., burns 300 calories an hour, which means you lose a pound ever twelve days or just over thirty pounds a year if you walk every day.

Apart from spading or other heavy manual work, the only other common exercises which promote significant weight loss are brisk bicycling and reasonably fast tennis, either of which burns approximately 450 calories per hour. Golf, with or without a cart, and such mild exercises as bowling, are hardly worth consideration. Regular exercise not only burns off excess poundage but also tones up the entire body, accelerates toxin elimination, and helps restore metabolism and the ACC level to normal. Exercise does not increase appetite or hunger. It is an essential part of any holistic weight loss program.

If fasting solely for weight loss, you may safely exercise during a five-day fast to speed up weight loss and to maintain muscle tone. Moderately long, brisk walks are probably the best exercise while fasting. Authorities suggest avoiding any jerky movements that might cause dizziness. If you are alternating five-day fasts with periods of eating, you can take longer walks while eating, or even jog or swim if you are in shape.

The typical American male consumes 2,400-4,500 calories per day. For the average 160-pound man who does not exercise, anything over 2,400 calories per day merely adds fat. To burn over 3,000 calories daily without adding weight, a 160-pound man would have to row, jog, or swim for one hour. Since few men perform such exercise, it all adds up to a huge problem of excess poundage. Exactly how much exercise you should take to lose weight depends on your ability and physical condition. As a general rule, the more exercise the better. If you walk briskly for two hours per day, you can burn off a pound in six days and over sixty pounds in a year. Although exercise is so essential and beneficial, if you are not accustomed to regular exercise, you must proceed with caution. Before starting to exercise, you should study Chapter IX in detail.

How To Eat Your Pounds Away

Eating Hygienically means living exclusively on fresh, uncooked fruits, vegetables, nuts, and seeds. Numerous studies have shown that people who live on such a diet are almost never overweight. The reason given is the extremely high fiber content of the food. Whole grain cereals are also high in fiber.

When you eat a conventional meal, it takes ten minutes after the stomach is filled before the "full" signal is actually experienced. It is, therefore, very easy to overeat on conventional foods and to take in surplus calories. But a high fiber diet takes longer to eat and you feel full and satisfied after eating fewer fats and calories. Also, since fruits, vegetables, and nuts require a good deal of chewing, more saliva and gastric juices are produced, causing the fibers to swell and increase the sensation of fullness. Little spare room is left for high calorie foods. The studies also show that on a high fiber diet, you excrete more fat and enjoy almost entirely dependable regularity.

According to David Reuben, MD., author of *The Save Your LIFE Diet,* regardless of how much you eat, on a high fiber diet the body will automatically reach its optimum weight and remain there as long as you continue to eat high fiber foods. If you are overweight, a high fiber diet allows you to lose weight automatically. But at least 80 percent of the diet must be high in fiber. Adding bran to a conventional low residue diet will prevent constipation. But it does little to aid weight loss.

Hygienic food is also rather low in calories. According to Dr. Neil Solomon of Johns Hopkins Hospital, Baltimore, most metabolic disorders can be reversed naturally with a low calorie diet. Although Hygienic foods are relatively low in calories, they more than supply calorie needs. Fruits and starchy vegetables are a Hygienist's main source of calories. Most people mistakenly believe that starchy vegetables like potatoes, sweet potatoes, or turnips are extremely fattening. "Not so," says famed nutritionist Dr. Jean Mayer. "Potatoes are not fattening. They are relatively low in calories. It's the gravy and butter that adds enormously to the calories—and the saturated fats."

For example, one helping of baked potatoes has only 94 calories, fewer than an apple. But the same sized helping of French Fries has 274 calories and of potato chips 557. It's what people put on their potatoes that is fattening.

Although some Hygienists do eat raw potatoes, parsnips, turnips, and other starchy vegetables, many others prefer to lightly steam them. Granted some nutrients are lost. But steaming for only a few minutes at not over 180°F (82°C) imparts a crisp, fresh taste to these energy-filled vegetables that makes them attractive and pleasant to eat. Since starchy vegetables constitute only about 15 percent of a Hygienist's daily food, 85 percent of his diet is still fresh, uncooked, and brimming with nutrients.

Complex unrefined carbohydrates like fresh fruits and vegetables contain only a fraction of the fat found in meat and animal products. Fruit, on average, has one-third the calories of meat and green vegetables about one-eighth. Most fruits, such as apples, oranges, and bananas, contain only about 100 calories. All fruits, vegetables and whole grain cereals are complex carbohydrates, meaning that they must be broken down in the digestive system before their nutrients can be released and absorbed. This process can take from ten minutes with sweet fruits to as much as several hours for starchy vegetables.

When carbohydrates such as sugar or wheat are processed and refined, they are broken down into such simple sugars that they can be rapidly digested and absorbed. Sugar is absorbed so rapidly when eating ice cream, sweet pastries, or dessert foods that the triglyceride and cholesterol levels in the blood stream are catapulted upwards, and they remain elevated for several hours. During this period, the organism exhibits symptoms of both diabetes and hypoglycemia. Simple, refined carbohydrates also contain far more calories. Sugar and white bread convert readily into fat in the organism, and brown sugar, honey, and molasses are not any better.

In discussing carbohydrates, we must specify exactly what *kind* of carbohydrate we're talking about. The Hygienic diet is a high carbohydrate diet. Approximately 80 percent of Hygienic food is carbohydrate, 10 percent is protein, and up to 10 percent is fat. But these are all complex carbohydrates that filter into the bloodstream gradually without overloading it with sugars.

If for some reason you cannot fast, you can lose weight steadily on the juice or mono-fruit diets described in Chapter V. But with patience and with willingness to exercise, you can also lose weight simply through eating regular Hygienic foods. You should, of course, eliminate avocadoes and replace nuts with sprouted beans and grains and cooked soybeans. Exactly how much you will lose depends on your excess poundage, your metabolism, and your willingness to exercise. Joan R's. record of 1.5 pounds per week is probably typical.

One reason why most fad diets fail is because they are low fiber diets. They are also diets. And "diet" to most people means something they will eventually stray from. Although we have talked about a Hygienic "diet", vegetarian eating does not imply dieting. Except for going easy on avocadoes, nuts, and seeds till normal weight is reached, you can eat literally all you want of just about anything in the entire vegetable kingdom. Calories are never counted. Which means it is easy and pleasurable to stay with for the rest of your life.

A REMINDER: that no one should ever fast for more than five days without experienced professional supervision. Study Chapter V in detail before attempting any fast and carefully read the section "Who Should NOT Fast."

The Living Food Diet

The Royal Road to Health and Youth

Thirty years ago, a machinist's mate in the U.S. Navy lived in an environment which could only be described as biologically detrimental to human life. There was little chance for fresh air, exercise, or getting in touch with Nature. Fresh fruits and vegetables were rarely served, and the food was invariably overcooked and lifeless.

Richard J., was still only in his late twenties when, after serving a hitch as machinist's mate, he was diagnosed in April 1948 as suffering from malignant melanoma. Existence of this most deadly of skin cancers was confirmed by both X-ray and biopsy. An immediately operation was recommended and surgeons removed the entire right side of Richard's chest, leaving the bones covered only by a thin layer of skin and a scar seventeen inches long. Richard was told that he stood only one chance in two of surviving for five years.

Richard spent three months in hopsital recuperating. every few hours, he was given penicillin, with other medications in between. In July 1948, he was released with instructions to eat a well balanced diet and never to sunbathe.

Richard spent the next two months investigating alternate healing systems. But his condition did not improve. His life insurance company cancelled his policy. During a check-up at the hospital, more lumps were found. At this point, Richard lost all confidence in the ability of medicine to cure him.

In 1950, Richard began investigating health foods and the natural health field. He attended a lecture on Natural Hygiene. Almost immediately, he underwent a fast and adopted a strict Hygienic routine. Shortly afterwards, he was able to stop wearing the eyeglasses he had used for ten years.

For the first time in his life, Richard's diet consisted entirely of living foods. Every cell in the fresh, whole fruits, vegetables, nuts, and seeds that he ate was *alive*. Most of the fruits, nuts, and seeds that Richard ate, as well as such vegetables as potatoes, beans and peas, are capable of growing into living organisms if planted in the ground. Except for untreated whole grains, all other foods are lifeless.

After a few months on living foods, Richard felt much better, and when he applied again for life insurance, he was unconditionally accepted. At least once a year, he took a therapeutic fast. No further lumps appeared. He and his wife subsequently had four children, three born at home.

Richard's operation was twenty-nine years ago. Today, lean, suntanned, and athletic, Richard J., operates one of American's most successful Hygienic institutions. All the other patients who were with Richard in the hospital ward in 1948 have died. Richard believes that, in part at least, he owes his life to living foods.

Some of the advantages of eating only living foods have already been discussed in Chapter I. Other studies have revealed that eating leafy, green vegetables provides protection against several types of cancer. But science, at this point, is unable to identify the specific elements that only living foods contain. Thus the benefits of living versus dead foods can only be assessed empirically, by observing people whose diet consists largely of living foods and comparing them with others who live on conventional food, most of which is lifeless.

Although such factors as exercise and lifestyle tend to weigh the evidence in favor of living food eaters, any overview would find abundant evidence to support the superiority of living food. We have only to cite the robust good health and extremely long lives of the Abkhasians, Vilcabambans, and Hunzas, described in Chapter I. California's Seventh Day Adventists, especially those who eat a lot of leafy, green vegetables and plant protein, also live longer and enjoy a standard of health far superior to the American average. Virtually anyone who has faithfully practiced Natural Hygiene for several years is fitter and healthier than his peers and will outlive them—even though in some cases, a Hygienist may have an irreversible disease.

Nutritionists who recognize the benefits of the living element in foods sometimes classify it as "Unidentified Essential Nutrients." By observing how man functions in sickness and health over at least fifteen decades, Hygienists are convinced that since primitive man evolved on living foods, the human organism is capable of optimum health only when fed a diet of *live, raw vegetarian foods!*

Cooking is basically a method of partially predigesting food which otherwise we cannot eat. Hygienists have difficulty accepting the theory that man was intended to eat flesh foods when almost none can be eaten raw. And when eaten, they are responsible for a string of killer diseases.

A report released early in 1977 by the prestigious Worldwatch Institute of Washington D.C., concluded that an affluent diet high in meats, dairy products, and refined flours and sugar, has been tied to six of the ten leading causes of death in the U.S., including diabetes, heart disease, stroke, arteriosclerosis, cirrhosis of the liver, and several types of cancer. The report, which was prepared for the U.N. Environmental Program, added that diet may be related to as much as half of all cancers in women and a third of all cancer in men. Among the cancers linked to our affluent diet were cancer of the bowel, breast, and prostate. The Hygienic diet is the very antithesis of the affluent American diet, which is being almost universally condemned as the direct cause of so many degenerative diseases.

A few years ago, orthodox nutritionists considered vegetarianism as nutritionally inadequate. Yet at least half the world's population is vegetarian and among these people—mostly Orientals and Africans—such common American diseases as heart attacks and strokes, cancer, diabetes, hypertension, appendicitis, and colitis are relatively rare. Since then, vegetarianism has become more acceptable. In his syndicated column "Food For Thought," well-known nutritionist Dr. Jean Mayer on December 9, 1976, endorsed vegetarianism and said that, even if not lacto-ovo, a vegetarian diet can supply adequate nutrition.

While most Americans have become aware that rich, high-risk foods are undesirable, a tremendous amount of confusing and conflicting advice is available about nutrition, much of it emanating from sources with something to promote or sell. Much of the advice is erroneous and misleading. For example, the manufacture and sale of food supplements through healthfood stores and magazines is a multi-million dollar industry. Healthfood magazines are filled with articles and editorials extolling the benefits of the same vitamins and food supplements which are promoted in their advertising pages. As a result, millions of people flock to healthfood stores believing that they can buy their way to health with a bottle of lifeless vitamin pills or bran, rose hips, dolomite tablets, papaya enzymes, bonemeal, or brewer's yeast.

When Nobel Laureate Professor Linus Pauling recommended in 1970 that taking one gram of Vitamin C daily would reduce frequency of colds by 45 percent, and the total number of days of illness due to colds by 60 percent, this claim by such a respected authority was super sales copy for Vitamin C manufacturers. At the first sign of a cold, Professor Pauling recommended increasing the daily dosage to four grams—which implied even greater sales of Vitamin C.

Professor Pauling's theory aroused such controversy that Dr. Terence W. Anderson, of the University of Toronto's School of Hygiene, organized a series of extensive studies to test it out. After numerous studies on thousands of students during two winters, Dr. Anderson reported that Vitamin C did seem to reduce the severity of a cold and fever, chills, and muscle aches. It did also cause less time to be lost from work. But Vitamin C did little to reduce the frequency of colds or their duration. Moreover, the studies showed that, normally, any Vitamin C intake exceeding 120 milligrams per day created body saturation and the surplus was simply excreted.

You can obtain 120 milligrams of Vitamin C per day by eating two medium sized oranges or eight Brussel sprouts or one stalk of broccoli.

Reviewing the Anderson study, *Consumer Reports* magazine (February, 1976) concluded that: "A daily intake of 120 milligrams of Vitamin C might actually be more than the body needs for colds or otherwise. Meanwhile, Consumer's Union has seen no persuasive evidence that amounts about 120 milligrams offer any further advantage to cold sufferers." *Consumer's Reports* also pointed out that taking large amounts of Vitamin C over a prolonged period might pose side effects such as diarrhea, Vitamin B-12 deficiency, and possibly adverse effects on the kidneys of a fetus. The magazine concurs that certain diseases do raise body requirements to more than 120 milligrams per day. But the common cold is not one of these diseases.

As you might guess, none of this was reported in the healthfood press. Although some so-called "healthfood" stores do sell such worthwhile foods as organically grown dates and figs, as well as nuts and seeds, and seeds for sprouting, most are simply high-profit vitamin and supplement dispensaries. There are more "healthy" foods on the average supermarket produce counter than in the average healthfood store.

Nothing annoys a Hygienist more than to be told: "Oh, you're living on healthfoods. You must be a food faddist." Are the foods upon which man has subsisted for millena "healthfoods?" Are potatoes, carrots, celery, lettuce, almonds, and parsnips "fad foods?" The real faddists are undoubtedly those who eat such nutritionally worthless "foods" as instant mashed potatoes or frozen TV dinners.

Hygienists do not use food supplements or fad foods of any type. No vitamins, chelated minerals, beef bonemeal, kelp tablets, double garlic chlorophyll, dessicated whole liver, or any other supposed "miracle" supplement has any place in the Hygienic diet. Even though commercially grown fruits and vegetables may lack the same abundance of rich nutrients as organically grown produce, Hygienists agree with the Department of Agriculture that commercially grown produce still has sufficient essential nutrients to supply the human organism.

For those who eat a lifeless, conventional diet of highly processed foods and animal products, a genuine nutritional deficiency may exist. Anyone eating the conventional meat and potatoes diet may well be in need of supplements. Cigarette smokers, in particular, often have a deficiency of Vitamins A and C. But Hygienists claim they do not need supplements. Which is one reason why few people have ever become rich from Natural Hygiene.

How To Tell If Your Diet Is Deficient

Some people are turned off vegetarianism by critics who claim it is deficient in Vitamin B-12, certain minerals, and complete protein. Most of the criticism comes from well meaning but uninformed people who would not recognize a nutritionally deficient person if they saw one.

You can often recognize a long-term vitamin deficiency by these symptoms: Cracks and sores in the corners of the mouth, especially accompanied by redness in the eyes, often indicates a deficiency in B vitamins. Gum bleeding while brushing teeth, provided it is not due to pyorrhea or poor dental hygiene, may be due to an insufficiency of Vitamin C. Joint pains, other than arthritic, may indicate a deficiency of Vitamins B, C, or D. Difficulty in seeing in the dark, or in adjusting to night vision, is indicative of a deficiency of Vitamin A. So are frequent coughs, colds, sneezing, and other upper respiratory problems. Ridges or other change of appearance in the tongue, may indicate a deficiency of B complex vitamins.

Hair, skin, and nails require newly synthesized protein for growth and their condition is an immediate clue to protein deficiency. If cuts and abrasions heal quickly, and if one's hair and nails appear in good condition, this is a reassuring sign of ample protein supply.

As long as you show none of these symptoms, you can be fairly sure that your diet is well supplied with essential nutrients. Since green leafy vegetables, darker colored vegetables, nuts, and seeds are richer in vitamins and minerals than most animal-derived foods, it is unlikely that you will ever suffer a vitamin or mineral deficiency as long as you eat an adequate amount.

Some people turn to vegetarianism for ethical reasons, believing that an animal's life is as important to the animal as a human's life is to a human. Spearheading the movement are the Vegans, a non-violent organization of ethical vegetarians, many of whom are also Hygienists. Some vegetarians go even further and claim that since eating a vegetable usually kills the plant, they will eat only fruits, nuts, and seeds. The danger of fruitarianism is that vegetables are the richest source of vitamins and minerals. Strict fruitarians live entirely on fruit. At least six Hygienic practitioners warn that a diet consisting exclusively of fruit is nutritionally deficient and all concurred that they had never seen a really healthy fruitarian. Dr. Paavo Airola, President of the International Academy of Biological Medicine, reports that many women fruitarians cease to menstruate and that many males become impotent.

What Not To Eat

Hygienists do not eat any foods derived from nonvegetarian sources. This rules out all meats, seafood, fish, poultry, eggs, and dairy products. All foods must be absolutely fresh and alive, so that eliminates foods that are frozen, canned, pickled, or preserved in any way. Natural drying is the only acceptable way of preserving foods such as dates, figs, or beans, and even these are second choice. Hygienists do not eat sauces, ketchup, mayonnaise, or condiments of any kind, including salt, vinegar, mustard, or pepper. Such condiments are used only to mask the taste of unwholesome foods. If condiments are necessary, then there must be something seriously wrong with what you are eating.

All foods must also be whole and unfragmented, which eliminates processed and refined foods of any kind, including bread and sugar. Prepared fats and oils—whether animals or vegetable—are also *tabu,* as are milk and all sweeteners.

Because only herbivorous animals eat grasses and cereals—and primates are considered frugivorous—Hygienists believe that man is not well adapted to eat grains or cereals prepared from grains. In any case, most commercial breakfast-type cereals are unacceptable.

Hygienists also have a few preferences among fruits, nuts, vegetables, and seeds. Legumes, such as beans and peas, are usually eaten raw and only when taken fresh and green from the garden. Otherwise, they are eaten only when sprouted. Peanuts, which are also legumes, are not as popular as nuts. Spinach, which contains nitrates, is not eaten because the nitrates can become nitrosamines, a potent carcinogen, when digested. Sharp or peppery vegetables, such as garlic, onions, radishes, parsley, or watercress are also avoided. However, some Hygienists use them in small quantities to flavor a salad, provided they do not burn the tongue. But don't expect miracles from eating garlic or any other herb.

Since Hygienic food is rich in fruit and vegetable juices, most Hygienists do not drink a great deal. Pure water is the only acceptable drink. The idea of drinking plenty of water to flush out the kidneys is considered fallacious in Hygienic circles. As water may dilute digestive juices in the stomach, Hygienists do not drink with meals nor within twenty minutes of starting to eat or for an hour afterward.

Isn't a diet of living foods awfully monotonous and dull? Not really. Depending on season, you can choose at any one time from twelve to eighteen or more different kinds of common vegetables, six or more different kinds of fruit, twelve different kinds of nuts and seeds, and at least a dozen different kinds of sprouts. After a short fast, or even after a few days of eating only living foods, all desire for lifeless foods should disappear.

Personally, we couldn't be tempted to eat a steak or hamburger, a broiled Dover sole, a plate of raw oysters, a pizza, or a slice of homebaked apple pie smothered in rich cream, even if we were offered a substantial cash reward for doing so. We do use some whole grain cere-

135

als and dried legumes and fruit when backpacking or canoeing in the wilderness. But even these don't compare in taste with the three great salads that we normally eat on six days each week.

Hygienists eat all foods with the skins on if possible. Due to pesticide spraying, this us unwise with commercially raised foods. All supermarket fruits and produce should be peeled. Alternatively, the outer leaves of lettuce and similar items should be removed and the top cut off. Tomatoes should be briefly dipped in boiling water and peeled. All other commercially grown fruits and vegetables, especially berries or grapes, should be thoroughly washed to try and remove the pesticide residue.

Due to pesticide problems, most Hygienists eventually become gardeners and raise their own organically grown fruits and produce. But organically grown sprouts and salad greens can be raised at home thoroughout the year, even in an apartment or mobile home. Foods can be safely stored in a refrigerator but wilted foods are never eaten. Ideally, both food and water should be taken at room temperature.

Organically grown fruits and vegetables are often available in fruit and vegetable shops or healthfood stores, albeit at somewhat higher prices. Tests have shown that approximately 20 percent of organically grown food sold in healthfood stores is not chemical-free. Apples, we've found, are particularly susceptible to fraud. Most organically grown apples show worm holes on the skin and evidence of worm activity in the core. They also tend to be uneven in shape and size.

You can often buy organically grown apples straight from the tree by contacting people who own small home orchards or apple trees in which they have no interest. Each October, we buy bushels of organically grown Red Delicious apples at far below supermarket prices. Stored in an underground root cellar, they keep fresh for months. We also store carrots underground in boxes of sawdust as well as other types of root and vine vegetables from our garden. A covering of straw will keep many garden vegetables growing till past Christmas. Under wooden frames, celery will thrive outdoors till the temperatue drops below zero.

By scouting around, we also buy organically grown concord grapes, cherries, pears, and peaches from neighbors at a fraction of supermarket prices. In Northern Colorado, our garden produces an abundance of fresh, organic vegetables from late May until the end of December. We raise a variety of sprouts all year and in winter, we raise salad greens indoors. Using trays filled with one one inch of soil and compost, we grow delicious buckwheat lettuce, pumpkin, squash, and sunflower greens—all organic and ready to eat only seven days after planting.

We buy our nuts and seeds, uncooked and unsalted of course, from healthfood stores or graineries. Walnuts are often sold in supermarkets. If not available locally, these can be purchased by mail order from sources advertised in such magazines as *Prevention* or *Let's Live*. The remainder of our food comes from the fruit and produce sections of local supermarkets, food cooperatives, or roadside stands.

How Often Should You Eat?

Many Hygienists skip breakfast and eat only two meals a day. The reasoning is that during the first half of the night, until around 5 a.m., the organism is digesting and assimilating food and restoring cells as we sleep. From 5-11 a.m., the blood is charged with cellular wastes and impurities which must be excreted through the kidneys. Thus many people do not really feel hungry till around mid-morning. A large, rich breakfast is merely a habit that places a heavy strain on the entire organism. People living close to Nature frequently work out in the fields from dawn until 11 a.m., before they are hungry and ready to eat.

The first meal of the day is invariably a fruit meal. On the premise that the fewer different kinds of fruits one eats at a time, the fewer enzymes are required for digestion, strict Hygienists often limit breakfst to only two different fruits. Typically, breakfast might be a large piece of watermelon and half a canteloupe or honeydew melon. (Melons are never mixed with other fruits.) Or it might be a pound of peaches and a pound of pears. Other Hygienists prefer a greater variety of fruits and their first meal might include an apple, a pear, a peach, a banana, and half a pound of grapes.

Beginners may find such an amount of fruit overwhelming at first. This is because fruit contains fructose, a fairly simple sugar that in large quantities can raise blood sugar levels. A large amount of fruit juice has the same effect. The rise is only temporary. But in the beginning, try to linger over fruit meals and avoid eating too much, especially dried fruits. After a few weeks, you will become adjusted to eating fruits and your triglycerides level will remain more stable.

The second meal, eaten in the early or middle evening, typically consists of a large vegetable salad composed of two, three, four, or more vegetables. Here again, strict Hygienists prefer less variety. A leafy green vegetable is always the basic component and the other vegetables could be alfalfa and mung bean sprouts. Following this comes the protein course, consisting of about three ounces of assorted nuts, seeds, and, perhaps, other sprouted beans and grains. About twice a week, the protein course is replaced by a starch course, typically consisting of one or two large potatoes, a sweet potato and an ear or two of corn. Ideally, these are chewed raw. But in practice, many Hygienists steam them lightly, imparting a crisp texture and palatable taste.

If you prefer a three-meal routine, you can have both a protein and a starch course each day. Here is a typical Hygienic menu:

Breakfast: three to five different kinds of fruit such as a pear, apple, banana, several plums, and a peach.

Lunch: a medium-sized vegetable salad with a tomato followed by a protein course of nuts, seeds, sprouted beans, and possibly sprouted grains.

For proper digestion, at least four hours should elapse between each meal. We prefer the three-meal routine, because both protein and starch are supplied daily. While snacks are not encouraged, Hygienists often munch two or three oranges, sometimes in place of breakfast.

Two rules govern Hygienic eating. First, a salad is always the main course and it is always served first. Secondly, the bulk of any Hygienic diet should consist of vegetables, not fruits.

In place of seasoning, Hygienists enjoy the subtle tastes of the fruits and vegetables themselves. However, if you change over gradually from conventional to Hygienic eating, you may prefer a simple salad dressing during the transition period. A tasty but harmless one can be made by mixing one-third cup lemon juice with two-thirds cup olive oil. Add a tomato and whip in the blender.

Like the Abkhasians, Hygienists take their meals leisurely. Try to relax for at least twenty minutes before eating. Dinner often takes a full hour, allowing ample time to chew everything well. Chewing breaks up the high fiber food, ensalivating it, and exposing it to the digestive juices. Since about 25 percent of the body's blood and much of its energy are mobilized for digestion, it is advisable to avoid doing any physical or mental work for an hour after a standard-sized meal.

Try to eat only when calm, unhurried, rested, and unworried. Rather than eat when emotionally upset or fatigued, most Hygienists would prefer to skip a meal. It's also unwise to eat immediately after exercising or when in pain. But the most important advice is to eat only when hungry. Skip a meal if you're not. Too many people tend to eat for entertainment. If something tastes good, we tend to stuff ourselves. Many people eat at least twice as much as they need. Even though it's almost impossible to become bloated on a Hygienic diet, or to add weight, it's still sound advice not to eat more than you really need. Always try to leave the table feeling slightly hungry.

It may sound surprising but many Hygienists eat only twelve meals a week. The reason? They fast for one day and eat only two meals per day during the other six days.

No one guarantees anything, of course, but the results of eating living food can be quite startling. People often lose up to ten pounds in the first month and almost everyone feels a new exuberance, an exhilarating lightness, and an abundance of energy. Even without fasting, the body gradually cleanses itself and after a few weeks, many people find that their arthritis pains have disappeared.

Obtaining Complete Protein From Living Foods

Early Hygienists observed that people fared better and had fewer digestive problems when they ate all their proteins together at one meal. It took over a century for orthodox nutritionists to make the same discovery. Nowadays, it is called Protein Complementing.

Proteins, the building blocks of our cells and tissues, are created from twenty-two different amino acids, all found in foods. Given a variety of amino acids, the body can synthesize a total of fourteen of the total twenty-two amino acids it needs. The remaining eight, which it cannot produce, are called Essential Amino Acids (EAAs). They must be obtained directly from foods. For a protein meal to be complete, all eight EAAs must be present. Most animal-derived foods contain all eight, and all are necessary for optimum health.

But vegetarian foods are often lacking in several EAAs. For example, vegetables are deficient in methionine, phenylalanine and isoleucine—three of the EAAs. But Brazil nuts contain methionine and phenylalanine, and cashews contain, in addition, isoleucine, lysine and tryptophane. Thus by complementing vegetables with these nuts, the three EAAs missing from vegetables are supplied by the Brazils and cashews.

With proper complementing, all eight EAAs can come

from vegetables, sprouts, nuts and seeds alone. Ideally, we suggest a mixture of unhulled sesame seeds, sunflower seeds, and assorted nuts with a green salad containing plenty of bean sprouts. Brazils and cashews should figure prominently among the nuts.

All of these proteins should be eaten at the same meal, preferably once a day. Protein cannot be stored in the body, hence nutritionists recommend a fresh supply each day. If all eight EAAs are not present at the same meal, many of the other proteins cannot be utilized and they are wasted. If you cannot obtain all of the EAA-containing foods, cooked soybeans may be used instead. Whole rice, wheat germ, oatmeal, and buckwheat are also good protein sources. But since these acid-forming beans and cereals ferment when digested together with nuts, seeds, and vegetables, most Hygienists avoid them. Nonetheless, sprouted grains of all types may be used to complement other protein sources.

For best complementing, use a variety of protein-containing vegetarian foods. Emphasis is on variety, not quantity. Given an adequately complemented mixture, surprisingly little of the mix is needed for satisfactory nutrition. For instance, a 130-pound woman needs only 66 grams of vegetable protein (about 2.25 ounces) and a 160-pound man approximately 80 grams (about 2.75 ounces) per day. Studies have shown that the human organism requires a maximum of only .37 grams of animal protein or .51 grams of complete vegetable protein daily per pound of body weight. On this basis, you can calculate your own personal protein needs. (One ounce equals 28.35 grams.) By matching vetetarian foods with different protein contents, Hygienists enjoy a protein usability equivalent to meat protein.

Proper Food Combining Eliminates Digestive Problems

If you've ever wondered why your stomach and intestines growl and cause gas to form, it's because you've eaten too many varieties of food that don't mix well. Try eating an entire meal of boiled potatoes, for example. Chances are it will digest so calmly and quietly that you'll be unaware you've even eaten it. But add a steak, beans, bread, a glass of milk, and some apple pie á la mode, and your belly may become a battleground.

The reason is that some of these foods are incompatible. When mixed in the digestive tract, they require so many different enzymes and digestive juices that the whole mass interacts and ferments, causing gas, bloating, and acid indigestion.

To digest starch requires ptyalin, an alkaline medium which is initially secreted in the mouth while chewing. To digest protein requires hydrochloric acid, an acid medium. Naturally, when the two are eaten together, they neutralize each other. Instead of being digested, they ferment, causing belching and gas.

If you eat a starch before a protein, you will also have gas, because starch requires comparatively little hydrochloric acid while protein requires considerably more. But if you eat the protein before the starch, there will be just enough hydrochloric acid left over to digest the starch without a fuss.

To avoid all digestive problems, Hygienists have perfected a system for combining foods properly. For instance, fruits and vegetables require totally different enzymes. So the two are never eaten together. Melons will not combine with anything, so they are invariably eaten alone. Proper combination is essential to provide compatible raw food combinations and to prevent fermenting and gas.

Critics of combining claim there is no such thing as a purely protein food, a pure starch or a pure fat food. All foods contain elements of protein, fat, and carbohydrate. While this is true, digestion seems to depend on the predominence of one of these factors. Whichever factor predominates seems to govern the behavior of any food during digestion. Hence Hygienists eat meals that are predominantly fruit, protein, green vegetable, or starch.

For proper combining, Hygienists classify every vegetable, fruit, nut, and seed into one of several food groups. You can identify to exactly which food group any item belongs from the lists below. Fruits are divided into three groups: Sweet, Sub-Acid, and Acid. In addition to never combining fruits with vegetables, you should also never combine acid with sweet fruits or proteins with starches. Green vegetables combine well with proteins or with starches but never with both together. Sub-acid fruits combine moderately well with acid fruits or sweet fruits. Avocadoes and tomatoes combine well with green vegetables. Melons are always eaten alone and mixed only with other melons.

The diagram makes it easy to recognize which food groups are good and bad combinations. The lists below identify to which groups most common fruits, vegetables, nuts, and seeds belong.

Starches: artichoke, beets, chestnut, carrots, corn, Hubbard squash, jicama, parsnips, peas, potatoes, pumpkin, rutabaga, sweet potato, yam.

Protein: almonds, bean sprouts, cashews, coconut, grain sprouts, hazel nuts, pecans, pine nuts, pistachio nuts, sesame seeds, soy beans, sunflower seeds, walnuts.

Green vegetables: alfalfa sprouts, bamboo shoots, broccoli, Brussell sprouts, cabbage, carrots, cauliflower, celery, chard, collander, cucumber, eggplant, endive, kale, kohlrabi, lettuce, okra, onions, pepper, radish, rhubarb, spinach, squash, turnip, watercress.

Sweet-fruits: banana, dates, figs (dried), mango, papaya, persimmons, prunes, raisins, zapote.

Sub-acid fruits: apple, apricot, blackberry, blueberry, chirimoya, cherry, figs (fresh), gooseberry, grapes, huckleberry, nectarine, peach, pear, plum, quince, raspberry, sapodilla.

Acid-fruits: current, grapefruit, guava, kumquat, loganberry, lemon, lime, orange, pineapple, pomegranate, tomato, strawberry, tamarind, tangerine.

Others: peanuts, legumes, and cereals are considered to be 50/50 starch and protein.

You will find these same rules work with convention foods. Eat a green leafy salad with a plate of cooked starchy vegetables and you'll have no trouble. Add proteins like fatty meat, dairy foods, or nuts, and the combination can be explosive.

Organic Greens Without Gardening For Pennies A Day

By sprouting seeds at home, you can raise an abundance of fresh, organically grown salad greens throughout the year. All you need are a few wide-mouth Mason jars or similar crocks, a few yards of cheese cloth, a box of strong rubber bands, and an old baking pan. Just about any untreated whole grain, bean, or seed can be sprouted. Among the most popular are alfalfa, mung beans, lentils, lettuce, clever, fenugreek, and sunflower

Proper Food Combinations

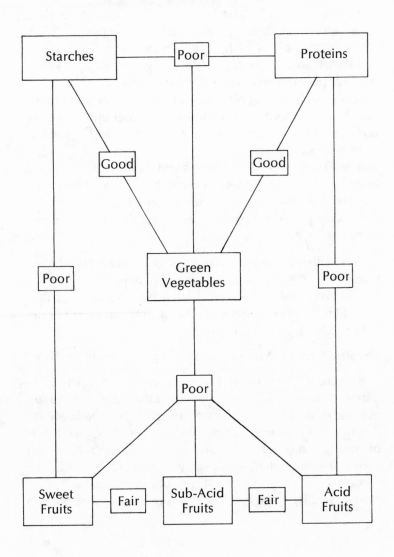

seeds; pinto and red kidney beans; black eyed peas; and wheat, rye, triticale, and other grains.

Most grains are ready for eating in only two days. Alfalfa, lentils, and fenugreek take about four days. Others may take a week. The process is simple. First, place one to six tablespoons of seeds in a jar. The smaller the seeds, the fewer you need. Alfalfa requires only one tablespoon, mung beans three tablespoons, lentils six. Fill the jar with lukewarm water. Then cover it with a piece of cheese cloth held in place with a rubber band. Soak the seeds overnight. Small seeds need only eight to ten hours of soaking, larger ones twelve to eighteen hours.

After soaking, drain the water. Then lean the jars against the edge of an old baking pan, facing down at an angle of about 30° so that the remainder of the water continues to drain into the pan while air can enter through the cheesecloth. Continue to rinse the seeds with cold water three times a day. Keep the jars in a warm place. Ideally, the temperature should stay between 68-72°F (20-22°C). If the temperature drops at night, growth may be slower. If during winter the air in your home becomes very dry, consider rinsing more frequently. During hot, humid weather, fewer rinsings may be needed.

In a few days, the seeds will sprout and fill the jar. Taste the sprouts at this point. If crisp and tender, they are ready for eating. Remove the cheesecloth and place the jar in the refrigerator. The longer you allow your sprouts to grow, the stronger the taste. Sprouted wheat, for example, is delicious when under an inch long but acquires a much stronger taste if allowed to continue growing. Even in the refrigerator, grains and beans will continue to grow.

Once in the refrigerator, your sprouts will remain fresh

and alive for at least a week. Meanwhile, you can raise another crop for the following week.

For best results, use high germination seeds sold in healthfood stores or advertised in organic gardening and food supplement magazines. When using large seeds, remove any that are broken, discolored, or shriveled. Each time you re-use the jars, they should be sterilized by soaking in hot water containing baking soda.

For variety, you can mix seeds with similar germination times, so that fenugreek, mung beans, and lentils can all grow together in the same jar. Most beans also sprout well together. Beans, by the way, prefer a slightly cooler temperature, especially in summer. Hygienists often sprout them for only two days indoors, then place them in the refrigerator for the final five days.

Seeds should be grown in daylight so that they fill with chlorophyll and turn a rich green. Commercially grown sprouts are usually raised in the dark and turn out a pallid white. Growers are also reported to use hormones or chemical fertilizers to stimulate growth. Though smaller, your own home-grown sprouts are far superior. For larger supplies of sprouts, you can shift to gallow jars. By growing six to eight different kinds of sprouts, you are assured a constant supply of pesticide-free greens at a fraction of the price of supermarket vegetables.

Indoor gardening goes beyond sprouting in that you can actually grow salad greens in soil. All you need are some trays one inch deep, some peat moss and soil, a plastic sheet, and some old newspapers. With this equipment, you can raise a rich supply of organically grown buckwheat lettuce; squash, sunflower or pumpkin greens; watercress; and whole grain and wheat grasses.

Any kind of watertight tray about one inch deep will

do. Begin by soaking the seeds for at least twelve hours. Next, place a thin layer of peat moss on the bottom of the tray and moisten. Fill the rest of the tray with rich, black soil. (If unavailable, mix together potting soil and organic fertilizer purchased at a garden store.) Drain the seeds and spread them thickly over the soil so that it is completely covered. The seeds can rest closely against each other. Do not press them into the soil. Moisten the whole tray again with water. Cover the tray with eight thicknesses of well-soaked newspaper. Finally, cover the whole thing with a sheet of plastic to keep in the moisture.

Seventy-two hours later, remove the plastic and newspapers. The seeds will be growing. Place the tray next to a window, preferably in sunlight. Moisten the tray twice daily for the next four days. By this time, the greens or wheat grass will be six to seven inches tall. To harvest, cut the stems with scissors about half an inch above the soil. Or, if you prefer, you can pull out the entire plant and eat the roots as well. Most roots are rich in Vitamin E.

Used soil can be placed in a large box and mixed with vegetable waste scraps to produce compost. When ready, you can then grow your seeds in compost instead of in fertilized potting soil. Compost formation can be speeded up by adding earthworms to the box.

For people with or without gardens, sprouting and indoor gardening can provide a wonderful assortment of organically grown salad greens at low cost and in all seasons.

How To Avoid Drinking Doctored Water

Save perhaps when performing strenuous work in hot

weather, most Hygienists drink relatively little water. They rely, instead, on obtaining fluids from fruits like watermelons that have a high water content. However, everyone needs water at times, particularly when fasting.

Almost all water from municipal supplies in America is heavily polluted and must be treated with chlorine to kill the bacteria. Various other chemicals are also added, including fluoride. The result is drinking water that often borders on being pathological.

According to Dr. Herbert Schwartz of Cumberland County College, Vineland, N.J.: "Cancer, heart trobule, and premature senility are conditions attributable to chlorine-treated water supplies. It has been shown that where people drink pure mountain water, pure and free of the chlorine found in big city water, they tend to live longer. I feel that if chlorine were now proposed for the first time to be used in drinking water, it would be banned by the FDA."

Dr. Schwartz isn't exaggerating. New Orleans water recently contained thirty-six organic compounds, of which three were toxic and three carcinogenic when tested on lab rats. Not surprisingly, New Orleans has the sixth highest rate in the U.S. for bladder cancer and urinary tract cancer and the third highest rate for kidney cancer.

Even water from mountain streams and rainwater is not completely pure. Both contain industrial pollutants and nuclear fallout which rain picks up in the atmosphere as it drops. The only way to obtain absolutely pure water nowadays is to purchase a stainless steel distiller and distill your own. In 1977, it cost about 12¢ a gallon to produce distilled water at home.

If your water is hard or mineralized, this is another

good reason for purchasing a distiller. Minerals in water often cannot be used by the organism and they can create harmful deposits such as calcium in the joints or kidney stones. In hard water areas, chemical water softeners are often used to leach out the calcium and magnesium in the water. In their place is left a high sodium content which can exacerbate high blood pressure. You should never drink water that has passed through a softener.

Many newcomers to Natural Hygiene ask: "What, besides water, can a Hygienist drink?" If you must have a beverage, fresh fruit juices are best. Otherwise, out of the entire catalog of beverages, stimulants, herb teas, beer, wines, and spirits, there is not a single drink that can be truly called safe. Many herb teas contain theine and astringents. If you want a hot drink, the least damaging is probably linden tea or carob.

How Hygienists Have Fun At Parties And Social Functions

Rich, high-risk foods and intoxicating drinks are commonly served at social functions. Since people equate food with love, they are offended if you don't accept it.

The way out of this dilemma is to accept it but to ask for an extra helping of vegetables. You can then eat the vegetables and leave the meat, eggs, seafood, or other high fat food.

Another way is to claim that your doctor has ordered you to stay away from all fats, animal protein, and stimulants. Most people equate the orders of a doctor with the word of the Almighty himself and will accept your statement without question.

When the service is buffet style, you can simply help

yourself to vegetables and skip all fats and animal foods. Instead of a cocktail, ask for a glass of water or fruit juice. Or just go out to the kitchen and help yourself to a glass of water. No one will know it is not gin or vodka on the rocks. Besides, you probably won't be the only one avoiding alcohol. Vegetarianism is so common in college towns nowadays that most party hostesses serve non-animal fare.

Custom and social values still dictate our eating and drinking habits. But chances are that no one will notice what you eat or drink, and you'll enjoy yourself far more than will the others engulfed in an alcoholic haze.

How To Ease Gradually Into Hygienic Foods

If you aren't quite ready to plunge into a diet composed entirely of raw, living foods, you can still make a giant step towards better health by compromisng. First, you cut out all the really high risk foods. And second, you add as many living vegetarian foods as you can.

All fried foods, fatty meats, and organ meats should be phased out at once along with ham, hamburgers, bacon, eggs, seafood, and all regular dairy products. In place of meat, you could use cod or haddock, two very complete protein foods low in fat. Alternatively, you can use low- or no-fat plain yogurt or cottage cheese. Don't forget that the average 130-pound woman needs only about two ounces of animal protein daily, the average 160-pound man less than three ounces. Eating more is wasteful and dangerous.

If you cannot yet face fruit for breakfast, try oatmeal or another whole grain cereal. They are best bought from a healthfood store or grainery rather than from a supermarket. Try to avoid any packaged cereal, even if whole grain, that contains sweeteners; most also contain unde-

152

sirable coconut oil. Gradually, you can add fruit to your oatmeal while gradually phasing out the oatmeal. It's not an ideal food combination, but it will suffice during the transition period.

Everyone probably eats a small salad with dinner. Keep increasing the size of the salad, while you add to the amount of cooked vegetables in the main course and decrease the amount of meat. If you keep using meat, but only the leanest cuts. Poultry and veal are less fattening than marbled meats. Yet all are actually unnecessary, and the sooner you phase out all animal protein, the better.

Coffee and soft drinks should be eliminated as soon as possible. Most soft drinks are filled with carbonated water and sugar, caffeine, phosphoric acid, and artificial coloring, flavor, and preservative. Phosphoric acid rapidly eats away the enamel on teeth and sugar causes decay. A tooth left in a cola drink overnight will have its enamel completely destroyed by morning.

The really dangerous foods to get rid of are all shortening, fats, and oils; most foods of animal origin; and refined flour and sugar. In their place, you can serve delicious bean or vegetable soups, healthfood store spaghetti, unhusked rice, sourdough bread, skimmed non-fat milk, and cheese made from skimmed non-fat milk such as baker's, farmer's, or Hoop cheese. None of these foods compare nutritionally with living vegetarian foods but they are far less hazardous to your health than the really high risk foods rich in fat, cholesterol, and refined carbohydrates.

Bake, broil, roast, steam, or stew instead of frying. And strive for freshness. Even if using non-vegetarian food, avoid anything canned, frozen, processed, or preserved.

In six weeks or less, you should be able to gradually

phase out all non-Hygienic foods and replace them with living foods. Or even if you never eat 100 percent Hygienically, your health will be greatly improved if you switch to low-risk foods.

Nine Small Meals Are Healthier Than Three Large Ones

During the 1976 Natural Hygiene Convention, Dr. Alec Burton of Australia stressed that the principles of Natural Hygiene are by no means final or rigid and that the movement is always open to beneficial new ideas. Of course, it takes time for a staid organization to accept such apparently radical concepts as yoga meditation or eating nine small meals a day instead of two or three large ones. But individual Hygienists are less conservative. Despite apparent conflict with basic Hygienic principles, some Hygienists have experimented with nine small meals a day and are reporting very satisfying results.

A number of studies have shown that most anthropoids, as well as primitive human populations, nibble small amounts of food at frequent intervals rather than eating two or three full meals a day. According to Dr. Grant Gwineup, a professor at the University of California at Irvine, when meal patterns are changed from standard meals to nibbling, blood fat levels promptly drop. Dr. Gwineup found that eating ten small meals a day relieves the heart from the stress of digestion and helps to prevent heart attacks.

Dr. Paul Fábry, a professor or at Prague University, studied 1,133 men aged sixty to sixty-four and found that coronary heart disease was more common among those who ate three or fewer meals each day (30.5 percent had heart attacks) than among those who consumed the same ration spread over five meals or more (only 20 percent had heart attacks).

Animal experiments have also borne out the fact that digesting heavy meals is stressful and that the stomach and intestines of both animals and humans who eat large meals have expanded by approximately 40 percent to cope with the excess load. As a result, large meal eaters are processing and storing almost twice as much fat and sugars as people who eat smaller and more frequent meals.

The highly successful life-extension program of the Longevity Research Institute at Santa Barbara, California, is based on eating nine meals a day instead of three. Each normal meal is divided into three and eaten at intervals of approximately ninety minutes throughout the day. Studies have shown that without reducing the intake of food, but merely by eating nine mini-meals a day instead of the regular three, overweight people tend to lose approximately two pounds per week. It takes only a few weeks on a mini-meal routine for cholesterol and triglycerides level to drop to normal.

For best results, eat regular Hygienic foods. Otherwise, avoid all foods high in fats, cholesterol, and refined carbohydrates. All foods should be high in fiber. If you can also reduce your total food intake by a couple of hundred calories per day, weight loss can be dramatic.

The orthodox Hygienic objection to small meals is that there is insufficient input of food to trigger release of the necessary enzymes for proper digestion. This may be true. But using another traditional Hygienic principle, that of observing results, it is becoming increasingly obvious that a mini-meal routine brings undeniable benefits which are greater than those accruing to people who eat only two or three times daily.

We've tried the nine-meal routine and we are so impressed that whenever possible, meaning most of the time, we divide our food into mini-meals. We are never hungry and never full. Gas, bloating, or indigestion is unknown. Meals are so light and digestion so constant that we can exercise almost immediately after eating instead of having to wait an hour. And we are delightfully free of the sudden influx of blood sugar that used to raise our fat levels after digesting a normal sized meal.

How To Prevent Cavities By Cleaning Your Teeth The Natural Way

Once you stop eating refined carbohydrates, tooth cavities should diminish. But by cleaning your teeth the natural way, you should be able to eliminate all future cavities entirely.

Most people make a great show of brushing vigorously with a wide, thick brush and lots of soapy white toothpaste. All this does is to jam food particles down into the gum line where they rot and provide nutrients for colonies of bacteria that cause plaque and decay. Ninety-eight per cent of all cavities occur at the gum line.

To clean teeth naturally, you need: a narrow ficus toothbrush, a roll of unwaxed dental floss, and if you have any bridges, a box of floss threaders. Floss is available in both standard and extra-fine gauges. Use extra-fine if the spaces between your teeth are small. Toothpaste is unnecessary.

You must first learn an entirely new brushing technique. For practice, imagine your thumbnail is a

156

tooth and the flesh below it is your gum. Place the bristles against the bottom of your thumbnail and wriggle the brush slightly back and forth so that the bristles grind into the "gumline." Don't brush back and forth. Impart a grinding motion to the bristles so that they grind and crush the tooth along its gumline, breaking up and destroying all food particles and bacteria colonies. Gradually move the brush along so that you cover an entire area of gumline.

Now try it in your mouth. Wet the brush and clean the front gumline of your upper front teeth, then the gumline in rear. Keep the brush wet and rinsed out. Go completely around your mouth, taking care not to miss the gumline around your four rear teeth.

Next, break off about eighteen inches of floss, and run it in the spaces between all of your teeth. Saw it back and forth, scraping the teeth on both sides and running the floss right down to the gumline. Give a quick, final brush around your gums, tongue, and other tooth surfaces to remove plaque. Then rinse out your mouth.

Clean your teeth after every meal. If you eat nine meals daily, rinse out your mouth after every meal and clean your teeth after every third meal.

If you have any bridges, each night insert the floss in a threader and clean out any apertures under your bridges.

A REMINDER: for proper nutrition, your diet should include more vegetables than fruits, especially raw leafy green vegetables. Except when fasting, your body also requires the proper amount of complete vegetable protein every day.

157

How to Regain The Legs and Lungs of Your Youth

At eighty-one, Ms. Eula Weaver of Santa Monica, California, had suffered for years from multiple disease symptoms such as intermittent claudication, angina, hypertension, advanced atherosclerosis, and arthritis.

Her circulation was so impaired that even in summer she wore gloves to keep warm. She could walk only two to three blocks at most, and often walking only fifty yards caused her calves to cramp. Her angina was severe enough to limit most activities. At seventy-five she was hospitalized for a myocardial infarction (heart attack) and at eighty-one she was treated for congestive heart failure.

She had been under medical treatment for fourteen years. Ms. Weaver was taking eight different medications, including Aldomet, Esidri, K-lyte, Nitroglycerine, Digoxin, Arlidin, Pro-Banthine, and aspirin. In 1970, Ms.

Weaver began following the life-extension program created by the Longevity Research Institute of Santa Barbara, California. The program is based on a low fat, low protein diet. Like the Hygienic diet, the LRI diet is also high in fiber and complex carbohydrates such as fruits, vegetables, and whole grain cereals, and allows no sugar, salt, coffee, or stimulants.

Coupled with this diet is a daily program of walking or jogging. Physical activity is encouraged throughout the day. Consistent with their capabilities, participants are urged to walk farther and faster and to constantly attempt hillier routes.

After six months on this routine, Ms. Weaver was able to walk seven blocks three times a day. After one year, she was able to stop taking all medications. By 1973, she was walking three miles, jogging a quarter mile, and riding ten miles a day on a stationary bicycle.

In June 1974, at age eighty-five, Ms. Weaver jogged 800 meters at the Senior Olympics Meet in Irvine, California. Next day, she ran 1,500 meters. Altogether in 1974-75, she won a total of four gold medals for running the 800 and 1,500 meter events.

In 1976 she was jogging one mile and riding a stationary bicycle fifteen miles daily. For good measure, she lifted weights twice a week. The amazing transformation of this eighty-one year old invalid into a trophy-winning, eighty-seven-year old athelete provides incontestible proof of the tremendous recuperative powers of exercise.

Granted that diet and all the other factors of the Hygienic lifestyle are absolutley essential. But in our personal opinion, regular and *abundant* daily exercise—not just ten or fifteen minutes of token activity—can contribute more to restoring health, mobilizing stamina and energy, losing weight, and adding years to life than any other single factor.

For centuries, man has been programmed to believe that strenuous physical work and labor will lower his status. This belief is still so widespread among all social classes everywhere that, given a choice, most people exert themselves as little as possible. Such a perverted attitude is tragic. Numerous studies, including the 1948-71 Framingham Study, have proved beyond doubt that among sedentary people, the death rate from heart disease is at least five times as high as among people who exercise regularly. Another study made in 1975 by James White of the University of Southern California in San Diego revealed that young adults who exercise regularly run only one-fourteenth the risk of dying from coronary, circulatory, or pulmonary disease as their inactive peers.

Literally hundreds of studies have shown that a rhythmic endurance exercise such as brisk walking, jogging, swimming, or bicycling, when practiced daily for an hour or longer, protects the heart and arteries, lowers cholesterol, pulse, blood pressure levels, and minimizes risk of *all* degernerative and infectious diseases. Older people who exercise regularly rarely suffer from osteoporosis, a disease which makes bones brittle and fragile. Abundant exercise aids the body in maintaining proper metabolism and in eliminating wastes and impurities.

According to Dr. William Z. Zuti, head of the exercise physiology laboratory at Kansas State University, exercise alone is the healthiest way to lose weight. Dr. Zuti's experiments have shown that dieting alone causes loss of both fat and lean muscle tissue. Through exercise alone, or through a combination of diet and exercise, you will lose only fatty tissue.

One pound of human body fat contains 3,500 calories. If you work off 500 calories a day in exercise, you can lose a pound a week without dieting. To do this, you need only play fast tennis or bicycle at 10 m.p.h. for one hour and seven minutes each day; jog or swim the crawl for fifty minutes; walk at 3.5 m.p.h. for one hundred minutes; or row a boat or rowing machine for forty-five minutes. Keep it up for a year and you've lost fifty-two pounds.

Overweight people do not become hungry after exercise. Obese people burn their surplus fat during exercise and do not become excessively hungry. People of normal weight do develop slightly larger appetites but only to replace the calories used in exercise.

Almost all Americans have atherosclerosis. But those who indulge in abundant and regular rhythmic endurance-type exercise develp a youthful elasticity in their arteries that makes them almost immune to heart attack or stroke. Anyone who walks, jogs, swims, or bicycles for an hour a day at least five times a week develops additional arteries in the heart and elsewhere. Existing arteries grow in diameter. Exercise alone does not always clear clogged arteries. But if maintained continuously, exercise will cause new blood vessels to grow around blockages and plaques.

Instead of paying $20,000 or more for a risky coronary by-pass operation—in which the by-pass itself frequently becomes clogged in under a year—through exercise and Hygienic eating, you can give yourself a new coronary by-pass entirely free of risk and at zero cost. This, of course, assumes you begin exercising while there is still time to reverse the condition. It also assumes that stress tests show that it is safe for you to start an exercise program. All this, of course, is exactly what is being accomplished by the program of the Longevity Research Institute.

While the challege of exercise causes the body to build new arteries, a diet low in fat and cholesterol can actually unclog arteries by shrinking the cholesterol plaques that are causing the blocks. A combination of exercise and diet, such as that endorsed by Natural Hygiene or the Longevity Research Institute, can provide dramatic results.

But perhaps the greatest advantage of exercising is the permanent "high" that results. A British medical team headed by Dr. Malcolm Carruthers, consulting pathologist at London's St. Mary's Hospital, recently identified the hormone, called Norepinephrine, which boosts the spirits after exercise. Any rhythmic exercise that raises the pulse rate will, in ten to twelve minutes, double the body's level of Norepinephrine, destroying depression and creating an optimistic feeling of wellbeing, confidence and optimism that lasts at least twenty-four hours.

Yes. Strenuous exercise can cause fibrillation or congestive heart failure in people with an insufficient supply of oxygen to the heart muscle. If you are overweight or suffer from any chronic disease or have the slightest reason to suspect that exercise may impose a risk to your health, you should consult a physician before starting to exercise. However, unless the doctor has a treadmill or knows how to examine your heart during and after exercise, such an examination maybe of little use.

Giving Yourself A Stronger Heart And Lungs

The best and least risky way to begin an exercise program is by walking. Not only is brisk walking one of the best forms of exercise but it is seldom, if ever, dangerous. Assuming you are in reasonably good health, you should commence a daily walking program *immediately*. Start very moderately and then, very gradually, begin to increase your distance and speed. While walking, get in tune with your body and "listen" to it.

It should be unnecessary to have to say this. But we've become so appallingly mechanical and artificial that we've lost the feeling of what life really is. The average American is so out of touch with his body that he must undergo an extensive physical examination on sophisticated equipment before he even dares to run for the bus. By listening to the subtle signals from your body you will learn far more than you will ever find out from a battery of medical tests.

This advice is not intended as a substitute for a heart examination made by a capable physician using a treadmill. It *is* intended to get your started on brisk walks immediately. When you are ready to advance to jogging, you will have ample time to arrange for a medical examination if you still think you should have one.

Brisk walking can provide all the exercise you will ever need. By walking a greater distance, you can obtain exactly the same training effect as jogging provides. For instance, walking six miles in one hour and forty-five minutes will provide approximately the same benefits as jogging three miles in thirty-six minutes.

Begin by walking a distance that is well within your capability. Then very gradually increase your speed and distance. Never reach the stage of over-exertion or fatigue. It may take weeks before you are ready to walk a mile. However, most healthy people become capable walkers in only three or four weeks.

Once you experience the wonderful feeling of well-being that stays with you all day after an hour or so of brisk walking, you may be ready to graduate to jogging—which will make you feel even better at this point, you may wish to arrange for a medical check up to ensure that it is safe for you to jog. As you progress from walking to jogging, the build-up must be *very* gradual. It may be several weeks before you are ready to jog half a mile. But even if you stay with walking, you'll start to feel better right away. So get started immediately. And do remember that, regardless of weather, *you must keep exercising every day!*

"You can run away from most of the pressures of modern living by jogging," advises Senator Proximire who, at sixty, runs five miles to work and back every day. "You must start by walking and ease into jogging very gradually over a period of months. But once you start, you'll feel better than you ever have in your life. After a year, you'll be a trained athlete, and regardless whether you're twenty-five or seventy-five you'll be in better condition than ninety per cent of the players in the National Football League. If you run five miles a day seven days a week, you'll look better, your eyes and skin will be clearer, you'll be serene and relaxed, inches will melt off your waist, and strength will come to your arms and legs."

If you can't run, keep on walking. Older women, especially, may prefer to walk. Aerobics expert Dr. Kenneth Cooper states that our aerobic capacity can be benefitted as much by walking as by running. But you must walk farther and for a longer time each day. Once you become conditioned, you must walk at a brisk pace. Ambling around a golf course does no good. "From the standpoint of heart and circulation, a sixty-five-year old woman who walks five or six miles a day is in better physical condition than many college athletes," concludes Senator Proxmire.

Is there added danger to starting to exercise in the later years? And should you begin exercising even if you've been inactive for years? "Lack of exercise early in life is no barrier to being active in the later years," reports Dr. Herbert de Vries, who works in exercise and aging research at the USC Gerontology Center, University of Southern California. Conducting an exercise program with 122 men averaging seventy years of age, Dr. de Vries found that those men with the least amount of previous activity were those who made the best progress. Another study done in 1975 by Kenneth H. Sidney of the University of Toronto with a group of Canadians aged over sixty revealed that in as little as seven weeks, exercise can restore the elderly to levels of fitness normally enjoyed by people ten to twenty years younger.

How can you tell if you are overdoing it? By "listening" to your body, of course. Your body will give you plenty of warning signals. A sure sign of over-exertion is a tightness or pain in the chest with severe breathlessness. You should also stop immediately if you experience nausea, dizziness, lightheadedness, or loss of muscle control.

After exercising, rest for exactly one minute, then take your pulse. If it registers over 130 beats per minute, you are definitely fatigued. Reduce your speed and distance, and do not increase again until your pulse registers under 130. If your pulse is close to 100, you are in good condition. Five minutes after exercise, your pulse should register 120 or less; ten minutes after exercise, your pulse should register 100 or less. If higher, you are fatigued.

Keep a close check on these signs and make sure you don't overdo it. To provide any real benefit to the heart and arteries, exercise should be sufficiently intense to bring on panting for at least six minutes. The longer you pant, the greater the benefit. This is why we recommend walking or jogging rather than calisthenics, yoga, or lifting weights.

Once you have a walking or jogging program going, you can beneficially warm up beforehand by doing a few preliminary exercises. Before jogging, we do these exercises: one minute of the yoga "Salute to the Sun"; one minute of sit-ups; as many push-ups as we can do; one minute of alternate walking and flat-footed jogging; and one minute of continuous flat-footed jogging. (You'll find the "Salute to the Sun" demonstrated with photos in many books on hatha yoga.) A gradual warm-up like this will prevent almost all knee and joint complications, torn ligaments and pulled muscles. After jogging, we walk for five minutes to relax gradually and allow the blood to get out of the legs and into the torso and head.

Swimming, bicycling, or fast tennis can be just as beneficial as walking or jogging. But you must move briskly on a bicycle. Keep pedalling at a brisk pace and don't stop to coast. If you use a ten speed, once you are in condition, you should travel at closer to fourteen m.p.h. than ten.

Once in condition, you should do something to keep

the rest of your body toned up. We suggest walking or running only five times a week and on say, Tuesdays and Fridays, alternate with a period of calisthenics. Use exercises that develop the trunk, chest, arms, and neck. Push-ups, sit-ups, toe-touching, bending, and stretching are ideal for keeping the upper body in shape.

In a book of this scope, space prevents us from describing exactly what exercises you should do. Instead, try your public library. Almost every library has a shelf of books on physical culture, each crammed with drawings and photos illustrating how to do a wide variety of exercises.

Most exercise equipment is a waste of money, especially if power-driven. Weights are helpful in toning and building muscles but are not essential. A simple rowing machine could be worth buying. Belts and other devices supposed to take off weight are valueless. If you wish to buy something, a quality ten-speed bicycle can be a sound investment. Before buying, make sure you can ride safely on local roads and highways, not just residential streets. If roads are narrow and lack paved shoulders, cycling may be dangerous. A stationary bicycle, or rollers for your ten-speed, may be better.

An aluminum canoe can provide good exercise. You could use it once or twice a week in place of calisthenics, and almost any small boat can be fitted with oarlocks and eight-foot oars and rowed. You don't have to buy a racing shell. Cross-country skis can provide lots of exercise if winter snows make running impractical.

Gardening could replace the twice weekly calisthenics. Provided you do all your spading and forking by hand, and keep your knees straight so that you bend down from the hips, gardening can provide magnificent exercise. We spurn any books or advice on how to make gardening easier. Using power-driven machines or gardening the "lazy man's way" simply robs us of the strenuous physical activity that is our birthright. Vigorous and abundant daily exercise is as necessary to our bodies as food, air, and water.

How To Banish Middle-aged Weariness And Fatigue

Literally hundreds of people we've talked with complain that they lack the energy to exercise. What they really mean is that they lack the energy because they *don't* exercise. Most people fail to understand that you must exercise first. When the challenge of exercise is placed on the body, the organism will mobilize the needed energy.

If you'd like the energy and stamina to make a brisk ten-mile walk without tiring, then you must first walk ten miles. After walking ten miles several times, your body learns to mobilize the energy for a ten-mile walk. Keep walking ten miles every day and in two or three weeks, a ten-mile hike will seem like nothing.

Of course, there's an easier way. You can progress in gradual steps. Begin by walking one mile. Next day, walk two miles. Then simply add a mile each day. By the tenth day, your body will be putting out all the energy you need to walk ten miles.

Anyone who begins a daily walking program and builds up to walking a brisk six miles every day will develop dependable stamina and energy. You will never again complain of feeling listless or tired.

If you need more strength and energy in your arms and upper body, start a program of calisthenics. Walk or jog one day, do calisthenics the next. You can build

168

stamina, strength, and energy in any muscle group or in any part of your body simply by challenging it with exercise. Begin very easily. Increase very gradually. Don't overdo it. Provided you eat and live Hygienically, in a surprisingly short time you'll double your strenth, build unbelievable stamina, and develop abundant energy.

The President's Council on Physical Fitness points out in its manual that if you force yourself to exercise moderately, your body will mobilize energy and eliminate chronic tiredness and fatigue, tension, and muscular aches and pains. No one who exercises regularly ever complains of feeling tired. People who walk or jog an hour a day soon find they can work all day without become fatigued. Most minor muscular aches and pains are due to weakness caused by lack of exercise. They disappear a few weeks after you begin a regular exercise routine.

Physical activity is also the best antidote for tension. Stress releases energy which tenses the muscles for a primitive "fight or flight" reaction. When neither is possible, the muscles simply remain tense, keeping the whole body uptight. But exercise rapidly works off the accumulated tension, leaving the entire body loose and relaxed.

Our own exercise program is based on an hour of rhythmic endurance exercise every other day. On days in between, we alternate an hour of hatha yoga postures and an hour of calisthenics. On our rhythmic endurance exercise days, we may alternatively swim for an hour, ride a bicycle for 2.5 hours or, on weekends, take an all-day hike, bike ride, or cross-country ski tour. Again on weekends, we may substitute for calisthenics a half or full day of gardening, or several hours of canoe paddling.

Hatha yoga is a system of bending and strethcing posi-
tions which can make your spine as flexible as a kitten's
and keep every limb and joint amazingly supple. Each
posture also stimulates an endocrine gland, thus toning
up your entire physical and nervous system.

By itself, yoga lacks the steady rhythmic exercise of
walking or running that benefits the cardiovascular system. When yoga was developed several thousands years
ago, peoples' lives were filled with walking and manual
exercise. Today, yoga must be supplemented. Plan to alternate days on which you do yoga with days on which
you walk, jog, swim, or bicycle.

The best way to learn postures, or *asanas,* is to join a
class. Since authentic yoga must be taught without profit,
classes are usually free or nominally priced.

How To Dramatically Lower Your Pulse Rate And Blood Pressure

The average American male has a resting pulse rate of
seventy-two per minute—the average woman six to eight
beats higher. While physicians consider such levels average, they are certainly not normal. Hygienists regard
such high pulse rates as pathological.

Anyone who eats plenty of raw vegetarian food and
walks or jogs several miles daily has a resting pulse rate
at least twenty beats per minute lower. Many active
Hygienic men have pulse rates as low as forty. Few
Hygienic women have pulse rates above fifty-six.

It has been amply demonstrated that a diet of raw, living foods lowers the pulse rate by approximately four
beats per minute. The remainder of the reduction is due
to regular daily rhythmic exercise.

To attain this kind of result—to really benefit both your pulmonary and cardiovascular systems—your exercise should cause your pulse rate to rise during activity to around 130 beats per minute for at least thirty minutes at least three times each week. Jogging, swimming, or brisk bicycling will accomplish this goal. If you walk, you must also move at a brisk pace and go for at least ninety minutes at least three times each week.

Exercise is also the surest way to cause your blood pressure to drop. Each month, the Longevity Research Institute reports on the blood pressure reductions achieved by its thirty-day class. Typically, one class of twenty-two people with an average blood pressure of 122/77 at the start dropped their average blood pressure to 114/66 after just thirty days of walking and eating a diet low in fat and protein. The average distance walked was 8.21 miles per day. One class member, who began on hypertensive drugs with a blood pressure of 146/80, was able to stop taking drugs and ended the session with a blood pressure of 110/60. The same group achieved a reduction in cholesterol levels of 24-33 percent and in triglycerides (blood fats) of 36 percent.

Exercise also makes it easier to stop smoking or drinking. Many a smoker who begins to walk or jog finds that, for the first time in years, he is really filling his lungs with pure, fresh air. The experience is so revealing that the desire to smoke often fades away. In a similar manner, the desire for alcohol may also vanish.

You don't have to go hiking all day on Saturday nor spend Sunday working in the garden—though the more activity you indulge in, the better you'll feel. The world's healthiest, longest-lived people are on the go all day, every day.

If you cannot find a place to exercise outdoors, you can run in place, skip rope, or ride a stationary bike. However, an environment in which you cannot find a park or open space where you can walk or run safely in unpolluted air is hardly fit for human habitation. You may want to consider that hundreds of thousands of people are moving out of the big, congested cities and finding exciting new jobs and healthful new lives in small, safe towns across the country.

You can increase your physical activity by observing these principles. Stand or pace instead of sitting. Walk up and down stairs instead of using an elevator. Park your car several blocks from your destination and walk the rest of the way. Take a 5 minute walk every 90 minutes throughout the day. Never use a machine if you can use muscle-power. Run in place whenever possible. Do as many errands as you can by bicycle or on foot. Keeping active at all times can burn off a surprising number of calories. Standing up burns ten calories an hour more than sitting.

Sunbathing Gives You Extra Vitamin D

By exercising outdoors, wearing only trunks or shorts and halter, you can also enjoy a beneficial sunbath. Sunshine is an essential factor in the synthesis of Vitamin D, necessary for the health of bones and teeth. It is produced on the skin after exposure to sunlight. For best results, you should not bathe in water for several hours after sunbathing.

Over-exposure to sunshine can also cause skin cancer. Thus, in summer, you should limit sunbathing to the hours before ten and after two. Don't use sun lotion or sunglasses, if you can avoid them. A light tan is all you require. Thirty minutes exposure per day is ample.

Hygienists also avoid very hot or very cold baths. And they find no use for soaps, deodorants, skin cleaners, lotions, cosmetics, shampoos, or shaving creams. Get rid of all sprays and disinfectants, and keep your rooms free of dust and tobacco smoke.

Easy Exercises That Improve Your Eyesight

Every morning before breakfast, David Stry, who runs the Villa Vegetariana resort and Hygienic institution at Cuernavaca, Mexico, leads guests on a series of routines designed to exercise just about every one of the 700 different muscles in the body. Among these is an invaluable series of eye exercises. After two weeks, one guest told us that he could read fine print in the newspaper for the first time in seven years. Frankly, we found the eye exercises alone worth the entire cost of our stay.

David's system is based on exercising the muscles that move the eyes. Without exercises, the muscles atrophy and tension makes them rigid. As a result, the eyeball becomes distended and sight deteriorates. Viktor Engels, a Hygienist who began doing the same exercises at age seventy-four, soon regained normal vision. Today, he has not worn glasses for almost ten years.

To do the exercises, sit or stand outdoors; if this isn't possible, sit or stand indoors facing a window.

Exercise 1: Close the eyes and face the sun. Cup the palms of the hands over the eyes for five seconds so that you see black. With the eyelids closed, remove the hands and face the sun for five seconds. Then, for just a split second, open and close the eyes. If the sun is obscured by cloud, you can keep the eyes open slightly longer. The idea is to very briefly expose the pupil to full sunlight without causing damage. This exercise causes the iris to alternately open and then close as it reacts to light and dark.

For the remaining exercises, face away from the sun.

Exercise 2: Look diagonally upwards and to your left as high as possible, then diagonally down and to your right as low as possible. Then back up and to your left. Repeat ten times. Next, start diagonally high and to your right and repeat ten times in the opposite direction. Feel the eye muscles stretching as far as possible.

Next, look straight up, then straight down, and straight back up. Repeat ten times. Finally, look to your extreme right, then to your extreme left, and back to your extreme right. Repeat ten times.

Exercise 3: Look straight up. Now roll the eyes gradually around in a wide, clockwise circle. Make the circle as wide as possible. Repeat ten times. Then revolve the eyes ten times in the opposite direction. While rolling, stretch the muscles as much as possible.

Exercise 4: Place your right index finger on the bridge of your nose and gaze at it, cross-eyed, for twenty seconds. Move your finger to your chin and repeat. Then onto your forehead and repeat.

Exercise 5: Hold up the index fingers on both left and right hands. Spread them far apart so that you can just see both fingers with your peripheral vision. Hold for thirty seconds while you concentrate on seeing both fingers. Then place one hand overhead and the other near your lap or waist and repeat.

Exercise 6: Hold your right index fingertip about four inches in front of your nose. Locate a distant object as

174

far away as possible. Focus first on your fingertip, then on the distant object, and back to the fingertip. Wait till each is properly focused. Repeat twenty-five times.

Exercise 7: Close the eyes and squeeze the eye muscles for a few seconds. Meanwhile, rub the palms of the hands together to stimulate warmth. Relax the eye muscles and cup the palms over the eyes. Do not touch the eye. Hold for a full minute. The object is sensory images.

Repeat these exercises several times during the day whenever you have the opportunity. You may also do them indoors at night. Use a bright lamp instead of the sun.

10

Living a Low Stress Life
in a High Stress World

Irving H. was a human dynamo. From eight in the morning until eleven at night, weekends included, he worked feverishly to build up sales in his real estate agency. Although he was relatively fit to begin with, the constant stress of working against deadlines and time pressures began to take its toll. Irving's blood pressure rose, and he developed backaches and headaches. He began to overeat and put on weight. This intensified his anxiety about his health and his future security.

By age thirty-eight, Irving had a painful ulcer and was twenty-five pounds overweight. Despite taking a daily tranquilizer, business pressures only seemed to multiply, and he smoked and ate even more. His blood pressure reached 150/94.

His doctor told Irving that he was suffering from hypertension and that he must slow down or risk a serious ill-ness. The medications his doctor prescribed were relaxing, but they left Irving feeling like a wrung-out dishcloth. Irving was contemplating psychoanalysis when a friend recommended fasting.

Irving flew down to Villa Vegetariana in Mexico and fasted for twenty-one days. He stopped smoking, his blood pressure fell to 130/82, and he lost twenty-four pounds.

Irving learned that regular daily exercise could relieve the tension caused by business stress. But only a change of lifestyle and attitude could permanently reduce the damaging effects of stress.

Villa Vegetariana is perhaps more receptive to new ideas than some of the more conservative Hygienic institutions. Several times a week, a local yoga teacher taught meditation and relaxation techniques. He told Irving that our minds and bodies completely interact. Thoughts affect our bodies and imbalances in body chemistry affect our thoughts. It is not holistic to merely treat the body and ignore the mind.

The yoga instructor taught Irving a simple three-step relaxation technique that, in a few weeks, totally restructured his mental concepts and eliminated his compulsive drive to create security behind a fortress of money.

First, he showed Irving how, in under five minutes, he could completely relax both body and mind. From this stage, it was natural to move to the next step, which was yoga meditation. In a few brief minutes, this powerful technique tamed Irving's churning mind, replacing his ambitions about business and money with a detached peace and calm that lasted all day. This set the stage for the third step, in which Irving spent five to ten minutes visualizing himself in perfect health. In his mind, Irving pictured himself at his ideal weight: strong, filled with energy, and free of all worries and concern.

Back home, Irving found his life completely transformed. By living Hygienically, he was able to eat all he wanted without gaining weight. A brisk walk each day helped eliminate his ulcer, headaches, and backaches. And the yoga relaxation technique changed his entire personality. Instead of making money his foremost goal, health became Irving's number one priority. From being a chronic, uptight worrier, he became poised and relaxed.

Now, three years later, with his aches and pains gone, Irving has married and enjoys a relaxed, productive life. Despite devoting time each day to exercising and the yoga relaxation technique, Irving finds he actually has more free time than before. Through staying relaxed, he is able to accomplish far more than when he was rigid and tense.

How To Cultivate A Type B Personality

What Irving actually did was to change himself from a Type A to a Type B personality.

When Doctors Meyer Friedman and Ray Rosenman of Mount Zion Hospital Institute in San Francisco studied 3,500 men nearly two decades ago, they classified each man as a Type A or Type B.

Type A men were human dynamos—aggressive, ambitious, and obsessed with a profound sense of time urgency to "get things done." This caused the same type of stress that precipitated Irving's ill health.

Type B men took their time and never hurried. Yet, the

researchers found, these relaxed men often accomplished as much, or even more, than Type A's. Since these men were classified in 1960—at which time all of them were free of heart disease—the Type A's have suffered 2.5 times as many heart attacks as Type B's.

Stress is a biochemical reaction to an intense demand to adjust or adapt to changing circumstances or pressures. The circumstances that cause stress can be joyous as well as painful. Marriage, travel, or success can be equally as stressful as divorce, unemployment, or the death of a spouse. All create pressures which in turn arouse fear, greed, hostility, envy, or anxiety. These undesirable emotions trigger the glands to secret hormones that can destroy you.

Studies at the University of Rochester School of Medicine, and the State University of New York, have demonstrated that the body's immunological system functions best when a person is full of love, and that diseases, including cancer, commonly occur after a depressing emotional experience brought on by stress. Stored-up, emotional poisons eat away youth and bring on enervating fatigue. Atherosclerosis, coronary heart disease, hypertension, ulcers, and colitis have all been unmistakenly linked with emotional stress.

Stress, in itself, is not the killer. A person who is calm and detached can go through life unaffected by stress. But others react to stress with negative emotions. Negative emotions produce negative chemical changes in the body. It is a failure to release these pent-up negative emotions that cause damage. Fear or anger triggers the well-known "fight or flight" response when adrenalin is pumped into the bloodstream to prepare the body for an extreme physical emergency. The muscles are tensed to run for your life or to physically repel an attacker. Your blood is prepared to clot if you are wounded, and your muscles are tensed with speedily mobilized energy. If you could immediately run a hundred-meter dash or pummel the person or thing that is making you angry, you could release your pent-up tension and emotions, and you'd feel fine. But when you can do neither, the muscles stay tense and the body remains biochemically poised for a primitive physical response that is frequently impossible in our highly civilized society.

Societies and people who are emotionally uninhibited have low rates of cancer and other immune-related diseases. By contrast, people who become overwhelmed by stress—such as loss of money, home, job, or spouse—and who see everything as hopeless and decide to give up, are *very* frequent victims of cancer and other degenerative and infectious diseases.

Dr. Franz Alexander and associates at the University of Chicago Department of Psychoanalysis report finding that many arthritis sufferers have hostile or aggressive feelings which they bury. The same studies led this group of physicians to feel that many people with hypertension also bury their hostilities and tend to be resentful.

Dr. Harold Voth, of the Menninger Foundation, reported an overwhelming correlation between susceptibility to cancer and a melancholy, anxious disposition. Dr. Voth's study, which covered forty years, also found that many cancer patients suffer severe emotional stress within five years of the onset of the disease.

Undesirable emotions such as envy, hostility, and fear reduce the efficiency of the immunological system. When this happens, fewer antibodies are produced and resistance to infection weakens. Diseases like colds and pneumonia are commonly experienced after emotional stress. Considerable evidence also exists that cancer, arthritis, Graves' disease, bronchial asthma, multiple sclerosis, and myasthenia (a muscle disorder) are also immunological-deficiency diseases. Anyone prone to anger, irritation, envy, or anxiety has an increased chance of dying early.

Why Your Blood Pressure Is A Barometer Of How Long You Will Live

Tension is a form of toxemia that may surface in the digestive system with symptoms such as ulcers or colitis. Or, more commonly, it constricts the blood vessels and causes blood pressure to rise. The Framingham Study shows that even among moderately hypertensive people, with blood pressure readings of 160/95, risk of stroke was five times as great as in people with blood pressures below 140/90.

The average middle-aged American's blood pressure is probably 120/80. Physicians consider that any reading over 140/90 indicates elevated blood pressure and hypertension. The 1960-62 National Helath Survey indicated that 15 percent of the U.S. population suffers from definite hypertension (levels of 160/95 and over) and that another 15 percent have borderline hypertension (levels of 140/90 or over).

Frequency of hypertension increases with age. Below age fifty, it is more common in men; above fifty, it becomes more common in women. The Framingham and other studies have proved beyond doubt that hypertension surpasses even the cholesterol level as the most important risk factor in coronary heart disease.

High blood pressure shortens life. At age forty-five, a

man with a blood pressure of 150/100 can expect to die 11.5 years sooner than a man with a more normal pressure of 120/80. Insurance companies attach such significance to elevated blood pressure that they levy an extra premium on even mildly elevated blood pressure cases, sometimes as low as 150/80 or 130/93.

Hypertension can also be caused by cholesterol deposits and by cigarette smoking, two forms of toxemia which constrict arteries. But the principal cause of high blood pressure is tension caused by stress. Tension is another form of toxemia which also constricts the arteries and forces up blood pressure. While high blood pressure can cause damage to kidneys and other organs, it is merely a symptom of a deeper, underlying toxic condition. Threating hypertension with drugs is merely palliative. To remove it, you must remove the cause.

Job and marriage problems are frequently the most aggravating causes of stress. Studies have shown that at least 15-20 percent of U.S. workers complain that their jobs are repetitive and uninspiring, that their work provides no challege, no pride in the job, and no voice in decision making. Most job dissatisfaction is with assembly line work and clerical work on the lowest rungs of the ladder, and hypertension is much more common among lower echelon workers than among executives.

The nature of some jobs, such as that of airline traffic controller, also creates pressure-cooker tensions from which it may take hours to unwind. If your job is causing stress, consider making long range plans that will lead to a more creative job that utilizes your full capabilities. If the nature of your job is stressful, consider eventually switching to a more restful occupation.

Marriage relations are often easier to rectify. Making a

genuine effort to please a spouse is often far better than going through the trauma of divorce.

Meanwhile, Hygienic diet and exercise can reduce the ravages of stress. And by using the same three-step yoga relaxation technique taught to Irving, you may very well be able to eliminate all tension and emotional stress completely. We've divided the three-step technique into a series of easily-learned stages. Practice and perfect one stage before continuing to the next. The whole thing can become second nature in a single evening.

It's not essential to do all three steps every time. However, you will obtain better results from meditation and visualization if you are completely relaxed first. To carry out the techniques, you will need a quiet, private place where you will not be disturbed. This can be either indoors or out, weather permitting. Some people sunbathe while practicing their yoga techniques.

The Three-Step Yoga Technique
To Annihilate Tension And Achieve Emotional
Tranquillity

Step 1
How to Attain Deep and Lasting Relaxation

Stage 1: Total Physical Relaxation in 90 Seconds

Lie flat on your back, arms straight and with hands about eight inches from your sides. Support the head with a pillow of some kind.

Keeping it straight, raise the right leg till the ankle is six to eight inches off the floor. Inhale deeply. Tense every muscle in the entire limb including the calf, thigh, and all five toes. Hold the muscles fully tensed for as long as you can without discomfort. Usually this will be from five to ten seconds. Then release the muscles, and drop the leg gently to the floor. You can either exhale while tensing or release the breath when you let go. Repeat with the left leg.

Inhale again and tense both buttocks. Hold for as long as you comfortably can, five to ten seconds, and release.

Inhale, tense the abdomen, and release.

Make a fist with your right thumb and fingers. Inhale, tense the entire right shoulder, upper arm, forearm, and all five fingers. Hold and release. Repeat with the left arm.

Tense the neck muscles by pressing down on the back of the head and raising the back of the neck and shoulders off the ground. Hold and release. Roll the head loosely from side to side a few times.

Open your mouth as wide as possible, thrust out your tongue as far as you can, and look up as high as you are able. Hold for five seconds. Then immediately pull in your tongue, clamp your jaw shut tight, close your eyes, and screw up your face tightly. Hold your eye, jaw, and facial muscles tense for up to ten seconds. Release and relax.

Take six deep breaths. Remain loose and limp on the floor, breathing slowly in and out while you enjoy the sensation of deep, physical relaxation. What you have done, of course, is to burn up the energy that was keeping your muscles tense and uptight.

After practicing this routine a few times, you should be able to unwind physically in not more than ninety seconds. Should you feel yourself becoming tense during the day, you can use this technique even while sitting down or standing up.

After you've practiced it a few times and really appreciate the quick release from tension that results, you can practice tensing and releasing the entire body in fifteen seconds. Here's how.

Lie flat on your back. Raise you trunk 45° off the ground and hold the arms out in front, fists clenched. At the same time, raise both legs till the ankles are about a foot off the ground. Keep the legs straight.

Inhale deeply. Then tense every muscle in the body at once. Toes, calves, thighs, buttocks, abdomen, shoulders, upper arms, forearms, fingers, and neck. Screw up and tense the eyes, face, and jaw muscles. All at once. Hold as long as you comfortably can, for five to ten seconds. Then release the whole body, and drop limply and gently to the floor. Take six deep breaths as you enjoy being relaxed and entirely free of tension. With a little practice, the whole physical tensing and release can be done in a brief fifteen seconds.

Stage 2: Total Mental Relaxation In Ninety Seconds

If possible, stage 1 should preceded stage 2. Remain in the same prone position, physically relaxed and flat on your back.

Make a mental picture of a deep, transparent pool of water about twenty feet across and a hundred feet deep. The water has a greenish tinge but is so clear that you can see the white sandy bottom. Beautiful trees and flowers surround the pool. The surface is mirror-smooth and unruffled. It's a warm, peaceful summer day with a few tufts of white cloud dotting the clear blue sky overhead. Enjoy the roses, tulips, and hydrangeas that border the pool and inhale the fragrance of their blossoms. Do not visualize yourself in the scene nor any other people, birds, or animals.

Now picture a shiny, new dime being tossed into the center of the pool. Keep your eyes about two feet from the dime and follow it down as it rolls, twists, turns, and darts down into the translucent waters, shimmering and reflecting the sunlight from above. Twisting and flashing, the dime drops deeper and deeper into the still, silent depths. Watch it moving down, deeper and deeper into the profound stillness. After about forty seconds, it rests on the bottom, protected by a hundred feet of water from the stress and turmoil of the world outside.

Put your awareness on the dime, resting in utter silence on the still white sands in an underwater world of calm and tranquility. The restful calm and tranquil peace that your mind found and enjoyed on the pool bottom will stay with you.

With a little practice, you can complete this stage in ninety seconds. During the day, you can tame and calm your mind by carrying out this routine while sitting down. Now that your mind is calm and relaxed, you can reach a deeper stage of physical relaxation.

Stage 3: Deep Muscle Relaxation In Two Minutes

Remain in the same relaxed position, flat on the floor, head supported by a pillow. Breathe slowly and easily.

Place your awareness on the sole of the right foot. Silently, order your sole to relax. Move the awareness to your toes. Silently, order your toes to relax. Move your awareness to your ankle, and order it to relax. Move your awareness gradually up your right calf, knee, thigh, and buttocks. As you progress, silently repeat the order "Relax." Feel each area respond with the warm, heavy, limp sensation of deep relaxation.

When you have mentally relaxed the right leg from the

buttocks down, picture your right leg as a piece of tired, frayed, limp old rope, entirely free of even the slightest trace of stiffness. Imagine holding your leg at the buttock and shaking it out as if it were a piece of old rope. Your leg is now completely loose and relaxed, without a trace of stiffness or tension. Repeat with the left leg and "shake" it out.

Place your awareness on the abdomen muscle and relax it. Visualize it as a piece of old rope and "shake" the tension out of it also. Repeat the same procedure with your right shoulder, forearm, upper arm, hand and fingers. Mentally relax each muscle, then "shake" out your entire shoulder and arm. Repeat with the left arm.

Place your awareness on the base of your neck and mentally relax each of the muscles in your neck. Move gradually upwards, relaxing in turn your scalp, forehead, eyes, face, tongue, and jaws.

Place your awareness on the heart and relax it. Relax the lungs. Relax your digestive system.

At this point, silently tell yourself: "My entire body and mind are deeply and totally relaxed. My whole body feels warm, heavy, loose, and relaxed. My body feels so heavy, it is pressing into the floor. I feel warm and comfortable. I am as limp as a jellyfish. My mind is calm. My body is totally and deeply relaxed."

Take care not to hurry through this stage. You will experience a tremendous release from stress and tension, a profound joy in feeling both mentally and physically calm and relaxed. At this stage, your brain is responding to a slow alpha rhythm and you are in a state of deep suggestibility.

During the day, it is possible to attain a similar state of deep relaxation while seated in a chair.

Allowing ninety seconds to relax the body, ninety more to relax the mind, and an additional two minutes for deep muscle relaxation, you should easily be able to run through all three stages of Step 1 and reach a state of total relaxation in five minutes.

Now you can go directly into meditation (Step 2) or Visualization (Step 3).

Step 2
A Five-Minute Meditation Exercise That Can Banish All Fear And Anxiety

Numerous studies have demonstrated that meditation, transcendental or otherwise, can eliminate almost all fear and anxiety. As a result, people who meditate regularly usually find that their diastolic blood pressure drops two to four points and sometimes as much as 10-12 percent.

In stage 2 of the previous Step, we described a simple technique that tamed the tumultuous churning of the mind. This same method can actually be used to enter meditation, a relaxed mental state in which all thoughts are stilled and perfect peace and calm attained.

In Yoga, meditation is achieved by distracting the mind with some senseless task such as repeating a word or "watching" one's breath, so that the restless flow of disturbing thoughts and worries is halted. With very little practice, it is easy to empty the mind completely of all thoughts. At this stage, you can experience a wonderfully restful condition completely free of such undesirable emotions as fear, hostility, envy, and anxiety and the disturbing thoughts they create. You will meditate best if you have already just practiced one or more stages of Step 1.

Sit cross-legged on the floor (in the yoga lotus position if you can); otherwise, sit on a chair. Place your awareness on your nostrils at the tip of your nose, and "watch" the breath as you inhale, then exhale. Concentrate on your breath. Each time you inhale, silently chant the word "Peace." Each time you exhale, chant "Calm." Keep watching the breath and chanting silently.

In a very short time, your brainwaves will drop into the relaxed alpha frequency, your breathing will become slow and shallow, and you will have entered meditation. At this point, you can cease chanting and watching the breath. Place the awareness on the center of the brain and just let things happen. Don't consciously try to think. If a thought or image intrudes, thrust it to one side. Your mind will remain comfortably blank and you will enjoy a level of calm and peace that you never thought possible.

After a few practice sessions, five minutes should allow you access to deep meditation. This is usually all that is required to banish fear and anxiety. Many people find meditation so pleasant that they meditate for a longer period. The longer you meditate, the better. Yogis call meditating "entering the silence." As you experience deeper and deeper meditation, both your psyche and your mind will desire it more and more. To ensure that this is possible, your subconscious will not permit the luxury of further fear or worry that might interfere with meditation.

Besides quieting fear and anxiety, and lowering blood pressure, meditation has other advantages. It improves mental alertness, work performance, perceptual ability, and develops self-discipline. It also reduces the desire for excitement through drugs, stimulants, and food and increases the desire to live and eat in harmony with Nature. Meditation also produces a deep condition of suggestibility, the ideal state in which to enter Step 3.

Step 3
How To Order Your Subconscious To Improve Your Health

The subconscious mind will attempt to carry out any order which it is given. When a hypnotist relaxes the body and mind and speaks directly to the subconscious, ordering a wart to disappear, the growth may vanish in just a day or two. The subconscious understands the spoken word. But it reacts most readily to picture language.

Visualizing yourself thirty pounds lighter, with better eyesight, jogging five miles, or enjoying raw food salads can work wonders in speeding your way towards better health. A few years ago, Dr. Cal O. Simonton, a cancer radiologist, taught a group of cancer patients how to meditate and then to picture their immunological systems destroying newly formed cancer cells. In a large group of men who had recently undergone cancer surgery, and then used Simonton's visualization technique, the mortality rate from recurring cancer was substantially reduced.

Dr. Simonton's method was so successful that it was recently being used at the Center for the Healting Arts in Los Angeles. Using a holistic approach modelled after Simonton's method, patients relax deeply and visualize their body's white cells on a search and destroy mission to annihilate any further cancer growths the moment they appear. Psychiatrist Gerald Jamponsky is also reported using hypnotic-meditative tehcniques adapted

190

from Simonton's method at the Center for Attitudinal Healing in Tiburon, California.

You must mentally picture whatever it is that you wish your body to do. To motivate your subconscious to cause your body to lose weight, you should visualize yourself as already thin. See yourself as able to jog along an ocean beach, legs and arms moving freely now they are devoid of surplus weight. Visualize the delicious smells and tastes of a large fruit salad that will replace the greasy plate of ham and eggs that you eat for breakfast at present.

Picture your reasons for wanting to be come slim—to lure a lover or reduce risk of degenerative disease—and review them in pictures each time you do the visualization technique. Just exactly what you will visualize depends on your goal. If you have a particularly stubborn condition of anxiety, you might use visualization to back up your meditation. You could picture yourself enjoying life now instead of wasting time worrying about possible future risks over which you have no control. Picture yourself simply giving up worrying.

Visualize your fears coming true. The bank you have your money in folds. You lose it all. So what? Health, not money, is your most precious possession. Picture yourself worrying and then realize how futile it is. Realize that worrying won't change a thing. A few examples like this will reveal to your subconscious the absurdity of worrying about things you cannot change.

Action is the positive answer to what is worrying you. If you are concerned about the possibility of a heart attack because you are a heavy cigarette smoker, picture yourself as a healthy non-smoker. Picture the vivid tastes and smells you will experience once you are free of tobacco. Picture your lungs, sweet and clear of foul smoke and tar deposits, effortlessly inhaling pure, fresh air. Picture yourself hiking easily up a mountain, inhaling the rich fragrance of alpine flowers while the sounds of a babbling stream tinkle in your ears.

Perhaps the strongest weapon in the entire arsenal of visualization is the demonstrated ability of the subconscious to strengthen the immunological system. An important part of the this system consists of aggressive white cells which are produced in the narrow of the longer bones and patrol the blood stream and tissues, seeking out and destroying invading virus and bacteria. Since body cells which become cancerous are also recognized as foreign, they are also attacked and destroyed. In this way, any cancerous cells which appear in our bodies are destroyed almost immediately, before they have a chance to divide and grow.

One caution: though meditation and visualization can apparently improve the efficiency of your immunological system, making it a much more potent defense against all kinds of infectious and immuno-deficiency diseases, it should not be relied upon alone to reverse cancer. In almost all cases where it has been successful with cancer, the patient has already received medical treatment for cancer. We do believe that, after cancer surgery, it can be a valuable tool in preventing recurrence of cancer.

Nonetheless, Alfred A. Barrios, Ph. D., and William S. Kroger, M.D., authors of "Psychological Variables and the Immunological Response; a New Approach to the Treatment of Cancer," in the 1975-76 *Journal of Holistic Health,* report that: "Both present authors have communicated with a number of doctors who have privately confided that they have brought about relatively permanent cures of cancer through hypnosis, but who would not make such claims public because they feared the reaction of their peers."

The process of hypnosis is virtually identical with that of meditation and visualization.

In his book *Relief Without Drugs*, Dr. Ainslie Meares, a noted Australian physician, describes how emptying the mind of all thoughts by meditation helps the body reestablish its immunological defenses.

Dr Meares cites the case of Mrs. Peggy Wells, a fifty-year old Australian woman who was dying of cancer of the stomach, spine, and breasts when he instructed her in the art of meditation. Mrs. Wells' condition was confirmed by Dr. Nigel Gray, a tumor specialist of the Victoria Anti-Cancer Clinic. Mrs. Wells' ovaries were removed and she underwent twenty-four radiation treatments. She also took Laetrile. But she refused surgery and her condition deteriorated. Yet ten months after commencing meditation, all signs of cancer had disappeared, and she was free of pain and well on the road to recovery.

So far, evidence proving the dependability of hypnosis, meditation, or visualization as therapies for cancer is insufficient. But the testimony we are able to quote does illustrate the tremendous power of the mind in organizing the body's defense mechanisms and in motivating the organism to attain almost any desired health goal.

Suppose, for example, that you have a staph infection in your left calf. The staph can be destroyed by your white cells. Invariably, when such an infection occurs, the white blood cell count rises as the organism produces them to battle the invading bacteria. Using Dr. Simonton's method, you would place your awareness on each of your larger bones, one by one, and visualize white cells pouring out of both ends. Spend a few moments visualizing the bones in the upper arms, forearms, thighs, and lower legs, each spewing out clouds of white cells from the ends. Then picture large numbers of white cells flowing through your bloodstream, moving through your body toward your left calf. As they arrive, they swarm to the infection like bees swarming into a hive. Each tiny cell has a mouth with which it attacks and destroys the invading staph cells. Picture hordes of newly arrived white cells attacking in waves until the staph is completely annihilated. Picture the sore on your leg subsiding and becoming well. The staph are all dead. Your white blood cell count returns to normal.

Visualizing for five or ten minutes once a day will normally motivate your subconscious into starting a long range program to improve your health. But in case of a critical infection, or the actual onset of a disease, you should visualize several times daily for as long as you can. (A Hygienist would also probably fast.)

Decide in advance what you are going to visualize and have a program ready before you begin to make mental pictures. To visualize, lie flat on your back, arms at your sides, head supported by a pillow. If you visualize immediately after meditating, no other preparations are required. You may also visualize after relaxing both mind and body through Step 1. Your brain waves must be in the quiet alpha state for mental pictures to make maximum impact on the highly suggestible subconscious.

You can intensify the power of mental pictures by repeating silent verbal suggestions to your subconscious. While picturing yourself as a non-smoker, you can silently repeat: "I hate smoking, Smoking ruins my smell and taste. Smoking is expensive. Smoking is threatening my life and health. I will stop smoking."

Don't visualize too many goals at one session. For best results, concentrate on a single problem at a time until it is solved.

Allowing five minutes for relaxation, five to ten minutes for meditation, and five to ten minutes for visualization, the entire three step process need occupy only fifteen to twenty-five minutes daily.

How To Survive The Built-In Stress Of Modern Living

Dr. Paul Dudley White first established that the best antidote to stress was to exercise vigorously and become physically tired every day.

You should also reduce commitments to a minimum. Avoid hectic tasks. Get out of civic and club responsibilities if they create time and deadline pressures. Allow yourself plenty of time to do everything. Use the time you save for exercise and the three-step yoga technique.

If your job is demanding, visualize yourself becoming emotionally detached from it. This means doing the job to the best of your ability without becoming personally involved. Set up an invisible wall between you and the pressures of the job so that regardless what happens at work, it doesn't affect you personally.

Best time for the three-step yoga technique is immediately before a meal. You'll emerge rejuvenated and relaxed and ready to eat.

Visualize yourself waking up five minutes before your

alarm is set. Almost invariably you'll find yourself waking five minutes earlier so that you don't have to jump out of bed immediately. Avoid starting the day in a rush, and allow yourself five extra minutes to unwind when you go to bed.

Rather than their bringing you freedom, you can become a slave to the many things you own. Mechanical or electronic machines can be particularly burdensome. CB Radios, TVs, stereos, automobiles, outboard motors, garden tractors, motor cycles, power mowers, power-driven tools, electric typewriters, and similar equipment is constantly breaking down. The more of them you own, the more time you must spend taking them to repair shops and hunting for spare parts. You can remove a great deal of stress by simplifying your life. Avoid owning sophisticated machines and appliances that you don't really need and that require expensive, time consuming repairs.

Plan one visualization session in which you forgive yourself for all the mistakes you've ever made. Forgive every person who may have hurt you in the past.

Take an occasional picture vacation. Visualize yourself at a quiet, beautiful vacation spot which revives pleasant sights, sounds, and memories. Picture yourself performing kind acts and good deeds. You'll emerge feeling confident, secure and optimistic.

If you've postponed becoming a Hygienist, visualize yourself taking the plunge and reaping all the health benefits. If you have a disease or condition that is reversible by natural methods, visualize yourself already restored to health. If you have arthritis, for example, visualize yourself entirely free of swelling and pain, running and jumping like a young deer. Since you've already read this book and have learned that Natural Hygiene offers a road back to health, your subconscious can automatically program you to take the Hygienic route at the first opportunity.

Six Ways To Lower Your Blood Pressure Without Drugs

The lower your blood pressure, the longer you will live. Most active centenarians have a blood pressure of 105/70 or less. Within limits, the lower your blood pressure, the better. Even if your blood pressure is considered normal, you'll be better off if you can lower it.

The first step in any do-it-yourself program to reduce blood pressure is to buy a home blood pressure kit consisting of a sphygmomanometer, inflatable cuff, and stethoscope. Complete kits are on sale in most drug stores and the price is usually equal to the cost of two brief visits to a doctor's office.

A single evening of practice is sufficient to master the art of taking your own, or someone else's, blood pressure. Blood pressure is recorded, for example, as 120/80 or 120 over 80. The first reading is the systolic pressure, measure when the heart contracts. The second reading is the diastolic pressure, measured when the heart relaxes between beats. A level of 120/80 is considered normal for most adults. With a kit, you can take your own blood pressure at any time without depending on a physician. And you can measure your own progress as you use the six steps described below.

Since high blood pressure is merely a symptom of an underlying toxemia, to reduce your blood pressure you must reduce the toxemia. Most hypertension can be reversed by a holistic approach that removes the six major causes of toxemia.

They are:

1. More Exercise. The benefits of exercise in reducing blood pressure were demonstrated by the famous Hansen-Nedde Study carried out in 1970 at the University of Vermont. A group of men with an average blood pressure of 168/92 trained for seven months in distance running, calisthenics, and other vigorous activities. At the end of this period, their average blood pressure had dropped to 134/75. The study proved that abundant daily exercise not only remedies high blood pressure but also prevents it.

If you haven't already done so, you should immediately begin a regular daily exercise program based on the recommednations in Chapter IX. Once you are in condition, you should walk at least six miles each day. Jogging, bicycling, or swimming are even more beneficial.

2. Eat a Low-Fat, Salt-Free Diet. Much high blood pressure is caused by cholesterol deposits which block the vascular system. The remedy here is to switch immediately to a diet low in fats and proteins and high in fruits and vegetables. You should change immediately to the Hygienic diet described in Chapter VIII. Plan to stay with it permanently. Salt should be eliminated from your diet.

3. Reduce Your Weight To The Ideal Level. Your ideal weight is probably a pound or two lower than the average weight for your height and build. Establish your ideal weight, then commence a fast, and continue until you reach your ideal weight. During the fast, your blood pressure will drop dramatically. Instructions for fasting to lose weight are given in Chapter VII.

4. Cut Out Stimulants. Cigarette smoking and drinking

tea, coffee, chocolate, cocoa, or cola drinks can raise your blood pressure. You can break dependency on these drugs by using the fasting method described in Chapter VI.

Another type of stimulant to eliminate is porno movies. Watching these movies creates an undesirable type of excitement that can send blood pressure soaring. Conversely, having sexual intercourse lowers blood pressure.

5. Reduce Stress. Plan to eliminate everything in your life that causes excessive pressures, You'll find an abundance of suggestions earlier in this chapter. A hot daily bath can help reduce tension and blood pressure.

6. Meditate and Visualize. In 1974, H. Benson and his associates studies hypertensive patients who practiced meditation for one month. During this period, their average systolic blood pressure dropped by seven points and their average diastolic pressure by four points. But the benefits continued only as long as the patients continued to meditate.

In our own experiments with visualization, we obtained better results by picturing ourselves as completely unworried, wound down and relaxed than we did by trying to picture our blood pressure actually falling. We obtained the best results by visualizing ourselves without a worry in the world, free of all enslaving possessions and demands, in a beautiful calm place far from tension and turmoil. If you can picture yourself in a similar Utopia, and repeat it every day, your blood pressure should drop by two to four points or more.

Make all six of these natural approaches a regular part of your life, and high blood pressure should become just a memory.

A Dependable Way To Enjoy Restful Sleep

If you live Hygienically, take plenty of exercise, and practice the three-step yoga technique described in this chapter, you should sleep like a six-year-old child. Should you still have trouble sleeping, the most likely cause is worry. Other reasons for insomnia include eating a meal high in fats just before bedtime, exercising just prior to bedtime, and failing to unwind before getting into bed.

To guarantee sleeping well, your bedroom should be quiet, dark and well-ventilated. The mattress should be fairly soft, the pillow substantial. (Foam rubber pillows are often too thin and yielding.) The temperature should be comfortable and the covers warm.

You'll sleep better if you go to bed fairly early. If you still have trouble sleeping, practice Step 1 of the three-step yoga technique immediately before dinner. Go through it again immediately before bedtime, and spend five minutes or so visualizing yourself falling into a deep, restful sleep.

About an hour before bedtime, relax in a warm tub. Then take a hot drink (linden or camomile tea, or carob) to bed with you. Another sleep-provoking step is to read a rather dull book before bedtime.

People who do not exercise often complain of insomnia. One reason is that they never become physically tired. Anyone who walks six miles a day, jogs, swims, or bicycles seldom fails to sleep. Insomniacs actually sleep more than they think they do. No one sleeps unbroken through the night. Sleep occurs in ninety-minute cycles. Most insomniacs simply wake up briefly every ninety minutes and then nap off again. In reality, most get all the sleep they need.

If you do wake in the middle of the night and cannot get back to sleep, practice Step 1 of the three-step yoga technique. In the unlikely event that you are still awake afterwards, spend several minutes visualizing yourself in a deep, undisturbed slumber.

Should you feel tired during the day, take a nap if you can. If napping is not convenient, close the eyes and shut out sound and light for a few minutes. A thirty-minute nap halfway through the day is a great re-juvenator, but you'll probably need a little less sleep at night.

11

How to Increase Your Sexual Drive and Vigor

And Maintain Sexual Potency Throughout Life

After studying 15,000 persons in the U.S.S.R. aged eighty and older, Professor Pitzkhelauri, a Soviet gerontologist, found that with rare exceptions, only married people reached a healthful old age. Many couples in Abkhasia have been married for seventy or more years. Professor Pitzkhelauri believes that marriage and a prolonged sex life are important factors in maintaining health to a ripe old age.

The principal cause of impotence in men is anxiety. But impotence is also caused by diabetes, endocrine gland disorders, excessive drinking, obesity, some prescription drugs, extreme fatigue, and prostatitis. These conditions are all symptoms of an underlying toxemia. Since Hygienists are almost entirely toxin-free, impotence among Hygienists is rare.

Excluding diabetes, impotence resulting from other toxemia-caused diseases responds well to fasting followed by strict Hygienic living, eating, and exercise. The files of every Hygienic institution list hundreds of cases of men who have regained sexual vigor through a short or moderate fast followed by close adherence to the Hygienic lifestyle.

Almost everyone could restore their sex drive by restoring their health. The two are synonymous. Get down to your ideal weight, cut out all stimulants, eat a living food diet, exercise regularly, and reduce anxiety by practicing the three-step yoga technique. In ninety-eight cases out of a hundred sexual potency will return.

If you are not diabetic, you can probably restore both health and sexual vigor without spending a penny and without having to leave home. Often enough, a do-it-yourself fast of four to five days to eliminate stimulants, followed by Hygienic eating and a regular exercise program, will restore the sex drive in as short a time as three weeks. If you are seriously overweight, a longer supervised fast may be necessary. You can also lose weight at home by fasting for five days every second week (see Chapter VII).

If you are diabetic, have your doctor place you on the medically approved low-fat, low-protein diet sponsored by the American Diabetes and American Dietetic Associations until you are no longer diabetic. After that, you can follow the Hygienic lifestyle.

Many common physician-prescribed and over-the-counter drugs have sex-negating side effects. Among them are painkillers including aspirin, tranquillizers, sleeping pills, and mood changing drugs. Anti-hypertensive drugs also have an adverse effect on male sex drive and performance, while anti-cholinergic drugs (used in treating peptic ulcers) impair sex response in both men and women. Alcohol also dampens the sexual urge. Non-essential drugs should be eliminated immediately, and maintenance drugs should be phased out with your doctor's cooperation. Ideally, you should then fast for a few days or longer before assuming the Hygienic lifestyle.

Hygienic publications often contain notices placed by older men and women who have regained sexual vigor by restoring their health, seeking to meet and marry a Hygienic partner. At Hygienic conventions, men and women in their seventies and eighties tirelessly dance till midnight, meet new partners, and make contacts that often lead to matrimony. These same healthfully vigorous people are out exercising again at 7:30 the following morning. They have learned that vigorous health and sexual vigor are identical.

Reducing An Enlarged Prostate The Natural Way

Prostatitis is inflammation of the prostate gland. The walnut-sized gland encircles the urinary tract immediately below the bladder. When it enlarges, it squeezes the tract, inhibiting urination and preventing the bladder from emptying properly. This may lead to bladder or urinary tract infections. It may also lead to impotence.

Prostatic enlargement is also invariably due to some form of toxemia. In non-vegetarian men over fifty, it is the primary genito-urinary disease. Medicine has no cure. The prostate is usually pared down surgically by a trans-urethral operation, a typical medical palliative which does nothing to remove the cause. Even when pared down to its original size, the prostate will enlarge again after a drinking bout or other dissipation.

By comparison, benign prostate enlargement often responds well to fasting. A five-day, do-it-yourself fast at home can often produce noticeable improvement. What the fast does, of course, is to allow the body to eliminate toxins and restore health. When toxemia is reduced, prostate enlargement usually subsides.

Most men with prostatis tend to be overweight, sedentary individuals with a long history of abusing the body. If you are in this category, you will obtain best results by undergoing a supervised fast at a Hygienic institution until all toxemia has been eliminated. This may take six weeks or more. Failing that, you can purify yourself at home through short do-it-yourself fasts coupled with Hygienic eating and exercise. Many men have completely recovered from prostatitis through Natural Hygiene, but recovery is permanent only as long as you follow the Hygienic lifestyle.

If you suspect prostate trouble, you should have a prostatic examination by a specialist to check for possible cancer. If your prostatic enlargement is benign, you need only observe the normal cautions described in the chapters on fasting, diet, and exercise.

Three Exercises That Will Help Your Prostate Shrink

Recovery from benign prostate enlargement can come about only from improved inner health. But several exercises seem to aid recovery, probably by stimulating the prostate area and by increasing blood flow and elimination of toxins. Allow several hours to elapse after eating before performing these exercises.

1. Yoga Mudra. Sit cross-legged on the floor (in the

yoga lotus position if you can). Place the hands behind the back clasping your left wrist with your right hand. Keeping the back as straight as possible, lean forward until your forehead touches the floor. Hold as long as you comfortably can. Repeat three times.

After some practice, you should be able to lock your feet into the lotus position. Place the left ankle on the right thigh. Cross the right leg over the left until the right ankle is resting on the left thigh. Or vice versa. Yoga Mudra is more effective this way.

2. Stomach Lift. Perform this exercise only on an empty stomach. Wear brief shorts or go naked so that you can observe your abdomen. Stand erect. Lean forward and place the hands on the thighs. Breathe deeply several times. Then exhale completely Force the air entirely out of the lungs. Pull in the abdomen. "Suck" it in, trying to draw your belly back against your spine.

Press your hands against your thighs. This will cause your abdomen muscles to rise and stand out. Hold as long as you comfortably can. Then let go and inhale several times. Repeat five times.

After you can perform this exercise confidently, try rolling the abdomen muscle from side to side by pressing first on one thigh and then on the other.

3. Leg Pressing. Make a loop with a piece of webbing about forty inches long. Lie on your back flat on the floor, legs straight, and slip the loop over both ankles. Raise the legs slightly off the floor and press them apart, pulling the loop taut. Press as hard as you can and hold for as long as is comfortable. Inhale before pressing and either exhale or hold the breath during the exercise. Repeat several times.

Performed daily or more often, these exercises often

prove extraordinarily beneficial while you are simultaneously purifying the body with fasting, living food, and regular exercise.

You can also help your prostate by visualizing it as small, healthy, and free of all disease—a small, horseshoe-shaped gland surrounding the urinary tract immediately below the bladder. Picture the prostate as enlarged, then slowly shrink it down to normal size (about the size of a walnut). Picture it glowing with good health. Picture your urine flowing freely and your bladder emptying completely. Picture your bladder as equally healthy and free of all infections and disease. Finally, picture yourself in vibrant good health with an athletic build.

One reason for prostatitis is repeated sexual stimulation without achieving a climax. Congestion results. The remedy is regular sexual intercourse. If this is not possible, masturbation once a week will prevent congestion.

If your impotence is caused by anxiety—by fear that you will be unable to perform sexually—it will usually respond to the three-step yoga technique described in Chapter X. Use the visualization period to picture yourself as a successful lover.

If you are not impotent, Hygienic living can double your vigor and sex drive. The closer you live to the Hygienic ideal, the greater the sexual vigor you will enjoy. Healthy men and women are often sexually active until well into their nineties. Some Abkhasian males have fathered children when aged over one hundred.

Lack of sex drive in women usually results from a premature slowdown in production of estrogen and other hormones. The cause is toxemia associated with overweight, mediocre physical health, and lack of fitness and energy. Because mind and body are completely inter-related, a woman who changes to the Hygienic lifestyle soon notices an increased interest in the opposite sex

The euphoria of well-being and the abundance of energy produced by good physical health stimulate the sex glands and can even break emotional blocks caused by disillusionment with past love affairs. Women must never forget that both mind and emotions respond im-mediately to an upgrading in physical health. An im-provement in physical health that makes you as lissome and fit as you were ten or fifteen years earlier not only makes you feel younger and more attractive but rekindles passions and desires of earlier years.

Since they stimulate the glands, hatha yoga postures are particularly helpful for women who have lost interest in sex. Yoga should be supplemented by regular rhythmic endurance exercises such as walking, jogging, swimming, or bicycling. Women have also found benefit in picturing themselves during visualization exercises as more passionate and more easily aroused.

By retaining sexual potency throughout life, Hygienic singles are frequently anxious to meet Hygienic partners of the opposite sex. Hygienic women are particularly in demand. By attending Hygienic conventions and joining your nearest American Natural Hygiene Society chapter, you may well meet other Hygienic singles. The Hygienic population is so small, and the proportion of sexually ac-tive Hygienists so much greater than in the general popu-lation, that a Hygienic single often stands an improved chance of finding a marriage partner through the Hygienic movement.

12

How to Add Twelve to Twenty Active, Productive Years to Your Life

"I'd sooner die young than grow old like that," is most peoples' reaction when they see a senile older person stooped over and shuffling along with stiff, faltering steps. While Leonard T.'s condition had not deteriorated quite this far, during his eighty-third year his senility did increase to the point where he was unable to communicate, walk by himself, or maintain toilet control.

At this stage, Leonard was enrolled in a month-long, live-in session at the Longevity Research Center at Santa Barbara, California. After thirty days on a low-fat diet, coupled with regular daily exercise, Leonard emerged as a completely new person. He regained his mental faculties to the point that he could carry on a spirited conversation. His ability to walk by himself returned, and he experienced a substantial return of other lost fuctions.

Fear of becoming senile discourages most Americans from any desire to prolong their lives. Yet gerontologists have proved that senility is both unnatural and unnecessary.

"The whole mass of our population is hung up on the idea that they'll come apart at the seems when they reach seventy," says Dr. John Thomas, eminent Harvard Medical School psychologist. "This fear of becoming frail and withdrawn and having to face years of senile decline, has caused most Americans to reject any desire to live to a ripe old age."

"Most cases of senility are not due to senility at all," comments Dr. Robert Butler, a Washington D.C. psychiatrist." Half of all Americans labelled senile are suffering from infections, anemia, malnutrition, excessive medication, or cardiovascular disease. Many doctors have a negative view of the elderly and don't care to take the time to diagnose their real problems."

The principal cause of senility is toxemia resulting from a diet high in fats and animal protein coupled with lack of exercise. Cholesterol deposits clog the blood vessels and cause atherosclerosis or hardening of the arteries. Atherosclerosis reduces blood circulation, cuts down the oxygen supply, inhibits the activity of the brain, nervous system, and limbs and produces the familiar doddering speech and slow, still movements.

As the LRI proved, once Leonard T. switched from the average American diet (42 percent of which is fat) to a diet of which only 10 percent was fat, he made a dramatic turnaround. The reduction in fat intake caused his cholesterol level to fall while exercise produced a new elasticity in his arteries. Leonard's atherosclerosis began to fade, and along with it went his senility.

As Leonard's case shows, if senility can be reversed by natural methods, it can also be prevented entirely. Thus it is not surprising to learn that Hygienists and most other vegetarians frequently reach their late eighties and nineties without a trace of senility. Anyone who lives Hygienically can outlive their life expectancy by at least a dozen years and in many cases, *by up to twenty years and more.*

What really counts is not your chronological age but your functional age. A Hygienist of eighty who is fit is as vigorous as an average American of fifty. We've met scores of Hygienists in their mid-eighties who had functional ages below forty. When we talk about Hygienists prolonging their life expectancy by twelve to twenty years, the years they are prolonging are their middle years, their years of greatest productivity. Through Natural Hygiene, you can actually double the number of your most productive years. Many Abkhasians and other longevous people retain youth well into their eighties.

The dramatic difference in lifespan between the average American and such people as Hygienists, vegetarians, yogis, Seventh Day Adventists, and the long-lived peoples of Abkhasia, Vilcabamba, and Hunza has so impressed scientists that around the world, gerontologists are busy plumbing the mysteries of growing old. So much has been learned that we already have the know-how for enjoying glowing good health for the maximum possible number of years.

The secrets of slowing the aging process and retaining youth are already available here and now. Don't look for any help from medical science. Most Americans mistakenly believe that our lifespan has increased phenomenally in the past fifty years. This is true only for infants. In

1970, the life expectancy of a newborn child was twenty years longer than in 1920. But by age five, a child's life expectancy was only ten years longer than in 1920. By age forty-five, an American male can expect to live only three years longer than in 1920. At age sixty, a man has life expectancy only two years longer than in 1789. Through safer childbirth and improved sanitation and hygiene, more people are attaining old age. *But they are not attaining older ages.*

Once you reach forty-five, all the great achievements of medical science have accomplished almost nothing toward increasing your life expectancy. By contrast, healthful living practices can do more to extend our lifespan than any drug or doctor.

Seven Simple Age Reversing Steps

For proof, we need only turn to a study directed by Ms. Nedra B. Belloc, a researcher in the Human Population Laboratory of the California State Department of Public Health at Berkeley. After sampling the living habits of 7,000 California adults over and eight-year period, the results of the study, published in the March 1973 issue of *Preventative Medicine,* proved statistically that by following seven simple health practices, middle-aged people can extend their lives by eleven to twelve years.

The most surprising thing about the seven health practices is that they are all well-known, simple, common-sense ways to take care of yourself. They are:

1. Stop smoking.
2. Take moderate exercise every day.
3. Keep your weight within reasonable limits.

4. Sleep at least seven hours each night but not over nine.
5. Don't skip breakfast, but avoid snacks.
6. Drink alcohol moderately, if at all. Drinks should not exceed two to three daily.
7. Maintain regular and moderate eating habits.

The exact number of years by which a person observing all seven habits can expect to outlive others observing fewer habits depends on age. At forty-five, a man practicing all seven habits can anticipate living a further 33.08 years as compared to only 21.63 years for a man practicing fewer than four of the habits. At age fifty-five, a man practicing all seven habits can anticipate living another 24.95 years compared to only 13.7 years for a man who practices fewer than four habits. This means that at fifty-five, a health-minded person has a life expectancy almost double that of a person who ignores his health.

With increasing age, the advantage gradually drops. But even at seventy-five, a health-oriented person can anticipate living four years longer than a person disinterested in health.

Dr. Ira Cisin, a professor of sociology at George Washington University, who helped research the study, said: "The study shows that your health and life are in your own hands, not in the hands of doctors."

Among other things, the study showed that a man of fifty-five who follows all seven habits is as healthy as the average American of twenty-five or thirty. Merely by following these seven steps, you can reduce your functional age by twenty-five to thirty years. The results of this study are telling us that we are really as old as our arteries, our spine, and our attitude.

213

Gerontologists have discovered that most of the symptoms and diseases of "old age" are not due to growing old at all but to such unhealthful habits as physical and mental inactivity, poor nutrition, overeating, and the ingesting of stimulants and drugs. Most Americans fail to attain their optimum lifespan because they commit slow, involuntary suicide by living a soft, artificial life in an overfed, overmedicated, and under-exercised society.

Yet numerous studies have shown that any normal man or woman has the innate capacity to remain healthy and active until well into the eighty decade of life. Some researchers claim that at least one American in two has the inborn potential to live healthfully for at least a hundred years.

Until quite recently, gerontologists believed each person had an optimum lifespan decided by sex and heredity. Statistics show women outlive men by roughly four years and that most long-lived people have long-lived parents and grandparents. For years it was assumed that longevity was inherited. Today more and more researchers believe that longevity is learned from parents and grandparents who practice healthful habits of living.

In societies where men are freed from the stress of deadlines and meeting bills, men tend to live as long as women. So even if you had short-lived ancestors, you may still have the potential to live one hundred healthful, happy years. The trick is to avoid the degenerative diseases and respiratory infections which kill off older Americans like flies. If you can avoid cardiovascular disease, cancer, high blood pressure, diabetes, and kidney or respiratory diseases, you should easily exceed your life expectancy by twelve to twenty years.

As we've documented in this book, Hygienists and

vegetarians in general have a far lower incidence of these diseases than the general public. Other things being equal, through living Hygienically you should anticipate a life expectancy at least twelve years longer than the average American of your age and sex.

Compared to the health-filled lifestyle of the average Hygienist, the seven health-giving practices just described are mild indeed. The seven practices fall far short of creating a lifestyle comparable to that of the long-lived peoples of Abkhasia, Hunza, and Vilcabamba. The seven habits fail to approximate the vigorous physical activity indulged in by most longevous people and to touch on such important factors as marriage and sex life, work and retirement, or disposition and attitude.

How to Make It to The Century Club

When reporters for the Social Security Administriation recently queried several hundred American centenarians, they found the same personality traits and living habits cropping up repeatedly. Virtually all of the centenarians:

—were even tempered, relaxed, happy, and unworried. They loved life and felt that regardless of what happened, everything would work out all right.

—worked hard all their lives.

—had long-lived parents and ancestors.

—ate a diet high in fruits, vegetables, and whole grain cereals and low in fats, meat, and animal-derived foods.

—ate lightly in amounts that kept their weight down.

—avoided cigarettes and drank very moderately, if at all.

—took abundant exercise every day.
Physical exertion was a way of life for almost all. They

played active games, danced, worked in their gardens and had lots of energetic fun.

Almost every centenarian we have met has been spry, trim, active, and nimble. In Abkhasia and other traditional centers of longevous people, older persons have always occupied a privileged and central position in an extensive multi-generation family. They continue to perform useful and essential work throughout their lives and are esteemed by everyone for their wisdom and experience. They head their families and make the decisions.

In Abkhasia, Hunza, and Vilcabamba, very few ever retire. In Abkhasia, Professor Pitzkhelauri found that when an older person lost his useful role in the community, he or she died soon afterwards.

This is exactly what happens, of course, when mandatory retirement at sixty-five is imposed upon us in our Western industrialized society. Each year, in the U.S. and other industrialized nations, enforced retirement suddenly renders millions of people useless, unemployed and often impoverished. Our artificial lifestyle imposes a role on us that almost inevitably hastens ill health and premature death.

Yet through Natural Hygiene, even the social death of enforced retirement can be transformed into the start of a healthful second career. Instead of spending meaningless years fishing or playing golf, most Hygienists graduate to an entirely new and satisfying life as an organic gardener or farmer. They never retire from this second career. By raising most of their own food, and by staying physically active and doing all their own maintenance and repairs, many Hygienists become almost self-sufficient and largely independent of our inflationary economy.

Whether or not you "retire" to the Garden Way of Life, if you are in your middle years, you can still extend your life expectancy by twelve to twenty years. Based on studies of the lifestyles of the world's longest-lived and most healthful peoples, here is an eighteen-point, anti-aging program designed to avoid the traps that rob us of our youth.

Eighteen Ways To Live Longer Without Growing Old

1. Think young, think health! In Abkhasia, most people expect to live to be over ninety. In the same way that we think of the average lifespan as being three-score years and ten, Abkhasians consider the average lifespan as being one hundred. Some gerontologists speculate that in our mortality-ridden society, we may be programming ourselves to a shorter lifespan.

Instead, visualize yourself as living a century. Make mental pictures of yourself in perfect health—now and in the future. Above all, have a purpose, a goal, a direction. Be going somewhere. Don't let mandatory retirement trap you into a life of inactivity and uninspired hobbies. Plan a second career based on the Garden Way of Living. Plan your retirement homestead with intent, ambition, and dedication.

2. Stay mentally and physically relaxed. Practice all three stages of Step 1 of the yoga relaxation technique (Chapter X) to ensure that you remain completely relaxed at all times.

3. Sleep at least eight hours each night. People who sleep eight hours a night have a lower mortality rate than those who sleep only seven hours and half the mortality rate of those who sleep for only six hours. You should not normally sleep for more than nine hours in each twenty-four. If you can't sleep more than six hours at night, try napping in the afternoon. See the section, "A dependable way to enjoy restful unbroken sleep," at the end of Chapter X. Never allow yourself to become over-taxed for more than one day.

4. Good emotions are the Rx for aging. Cultivate a Type B personality (see "How to cultivate a Type B personality" in Chapter X.) Roll with the punches instead of dissipating energy in trying to fight life. To live long and healthfully, avoid time pressures and deadline situations that pile up tensions and cause you to become uptight and overtaxed. Uncertainty and change can also lead to worry, doubt, and fear. So can such major life changes as marriage, divorce, retirement, a drop in financial status, assuming a large mortgage, or losing a love object. A cluster of such changes coming together can weaken the immunological system and trigger diseases.

You can avoid this risk by meditating regularly (Chapter X) and visualizing your body in top condition.

5. Keep your blood pressure low. Your blood pressure is a direct indication of how long you will live. The lower the pressure, the longer your life expectancy. Most people who live to be over ninety have blood pressures in the 105/70 range and lower. Yet in the U.S., one of every three adult males has hypertension or a tendency towards it. You can reduce your blood pressure yourself by natural methods. Look up "Six ways to lower your blood pressure without drugs" in Chapter X.

6. Work hard at a satisfying job. When Elliot Richardson was Secretary of HEW, he commissioned a study on work. The study showed that the highest indicator of longevity was work satisfaction. Being satisfied

218

with your job has a higher correlation with longer life than any other factor including general physical health. Among the longest-lived Americans are Justices of the U.S. Supreme Court, U.S. Senators, scientists, teachers, artists, musicians, organic farmers, and men in the learned professions, most of whom are free to continue working after sixty-five. Surveys show that people with higher education and thus more satisfying jobs have less stress and less hypertension, and they live longer than people of lower educational levels. The most healthful occupation is that of organic gardener or farmer.

If your work is satisfying and free of stress and you don't have to quit, postpone retirement as long as you can. If you are forced to retire, consider a new career based on the Garden Way of Life (Chapter XIII). Otherwise, try to fill at least part of your time with meaningful but tension-free work. If necessary, work without pay for a needy cause. Try to choose work where you make fullest use of your potentials and capabilities. Do the very best work that you can. Keep on working.

7. Eliminate all stimulants. Smokers have a death rate exactly double that of non-smokers, while heavy alcohol consumption produces a mortality rate two to three times that of the general population. Coffee drinking burdens the heart, interferes with sleep, raises blood pressure, and has been linked with cancer. Black tea, chocolate, cocoa, and cola drinks are almost as bad. Longevity seems unaffected by drinking only one or two mild alcoholic drinks per day. But no stimulant fills any real need and there is always the risk that, under stress, a mild drinker can become a heavy drinker. Chapter VI describes a painless way to phase out all stimulants through fasting.

8. Eliminate all drugs. The list of hazardous side effects and adverse reactions associated with every type of prescription and non-prescription drug grows daily. Many common maintenance drugs and medications have been linked with cancer, especially in women. Maintenance drugs, such as those used to control diabetes or hypertension provide a permanent source of revenue for drug manufacturers as well as a source of steady fees for the medical profession. If you are on a maintenance drug that is not absolutely essential, ask your doctor for permission to stop. If he won't cooperate, find another physician who will.

Almost invariably, maintenance drugs cause permanent damage to human organs. A short fast followed by a few weeks on a diet of raw fruits, vegetables, nuts, and seeds can do more for most ailments than a lifetime on drugs. Live Hygienically and you should never again require drugs or medication of any type.

9. Fast one day each week. Help roll back the years by going without food for twenty-four hours once each week. A one day fast gives your heart and digestive system a well-earned rest and almost guarantees freedom from any chronic digestive complaint. Even after a short fast, the body feels light, supple, and rejuvenated. Short, regular fasts keep the hair glistening, the eyes sparkling, and the skin free of blemishes. Look up "The wonderful benefits of a twenty-four hour fast" in Chapter V.

10. Exercise is the major antidote to aging. Invigorating daily exercise, which pumps oxygen to the brain, is the best insurance against senility as well as against heart attack stroke, atherosclerosis, hypertension, diabetes, arthritis, obesity, and osteoporosis. Dr. Herbert De Vries, Director of Exercise Physiology at the Andrus Gerontology Center, University of Southern California, found that when mature people take up a structured exercise program, many symptoms of aging are reversed. Through exercising a group of seventy-year-old men, Dr. De Vries found that their aerobic capacity increased by 29 percent, the same increase as in younger men who start to exercise. Studies have shown that an increase of 33 percent in aerobic capacity can prolong life by a decade or more. Regular daily rhythmic exercise can mean the difference between dying at seventy-five or living to be eighty-five or more.

People who exercise infrequently have a mortality rate twice that of people who exercise abundantly every day. Regular exercise can eliminate toxins, reduce tension, and even cut down on risk of cancer. A study in Japan revealed that mice which exercised regularly had a cancer rate 30 percent lower than sedentary mice. Scientists believe this is because exercise tones up the entire body including the immunological system.

But you must exercise continuously for a minimum of thirty-six minutes or more each day. See Chapter IX for details on planning your own exercise program.

You'll also look and feel a lot younger if you always walk erect and straight. Keep your head up and your shoulders back and down when you walk.

11. Eat small meals. That "gluttony kills more people than the sword" could be a reference to the common American practice of overeating and eating dangerously large meals. Digesting large meals, even Hygienic meals, places an added strain on the heart and raises triglycerides and blood sugar levels. You'll stay healthier and live longer if you cut down on meal size and always leave the table feeling slightly hungry. One way to accomplish this is to eat nine mini-meals daily instead of three large meals. See "Nine small meals are healthier than three large ones" in Chapter. VIII.

12. Eat a diet low in fats, cholesterol, animal protein, and refined carbohydrates. Dr. Beverly Winnikoff of the Rockefeller Foundation, reporting in 1977 on a two-year study of the eating and drinking habits of Americans, called for less salt, sugar, fat, refined foods, and animal protein in the national diet, and more foodstuffs containing crude fiber, particularly fresh fruits, vegetables, and whole grain cereals. "The way we eat is the way we die," Dr. Winnikoff told a conference of the nation's health leaders. "The way we eat sets the scene for our premature death."

In 1929, the average American consumed 400 pounds of fresh fruits and vegetables annually and under 100 pounds of processed foods. But in 1971, we used 300 pounds of processed foods and only 250 pounds of fresh fruits and vegetables. This change, Dr. Winnikoff believes, has forged the link between diet and killer diseases. Most Americans now eat a diet high in calories, fat, cholesterol, animal protein, and refined carbohydrates low in fiber.

Together with a decrease in exercise, this has resulted in an increasingly obese society. Approximately one third of Americans are obese to a degree which can shorten life. Obesity sets the stage for a number of lethal, degenerative diseases. Dr. Winnikoff also pointed out that high rates of meat consumption are associated with high rates of colon cancer; high rates of fat consumption with breast cancer; excessive sugar consumption with diabetes; and high use of salt with increased blood pressure.

By contrast, Hygienists who live almost exclusively on

raw, fresh fruits, vegetables, nuts, and seeds and almost entirely safe from the epidemic of degenerative diseases that today kills four of ever five Americans. Supporting the healthfulness of the Hygienic diet is a study recently made at the University of Buffalo by Dr. Saxton Graham which found that people who eat raw vegetables are significantly less likely to develop gastro-intestinal cancer.

Other studies have shown that the anti-oxidant properties of Vitamin E appear to be effective in extending the life of human cells. This has caused many people to begin taking Vitamin E in supplement form. Hygienists believe this is totally unnecessary, partly because larger doses of Vitamin E tend to increase blood pressure, and partly because the Hygienic diet is already rich in Vitamin E. Nuts, seeds, leafy green vegetables, beans and grains are all rich sources of natural Vitamin E. If you believe that Vitamin E can extend life, your best plan is to eat Hygienically. The Hygienic diet is described in Chapter VIII.

13. Keep down fat and body weight. Being moderately overweight is not as dangerous as smoking. But being 15 percent or more overweight does increase risk of heart attack, stroke, hypertension, diabetes, and other life-shortening disease. Anyone who is 30 percent or more overweight faces a serious risk of increased mortality. In all cases, natural reducing methods such as fasting, Hygienic eating, and exercise offer the safest and most rapid way to lose weight and keep it off. Chapter VII describes the Natural Hygiene way to become slim, slender, and attractive. (Chapters V, VIII, and IX are also required reading.)

Stop reducing whenever your weight drops a pound or two below the standard for your height and weight. The

Belloc study revealed that when weight drops 10 percent or more below the standard, the mortality risk begins to increase.

14. Drink pure water. The water supply of many U.S. cities is shockingly impure, especially where water is polluted by industrial poisons or agricultural pesticides and fertilizers. In Ohio cities on polluted Lake Erie and the Ohio River, cancer rates are 8 percent higher than in the rest of the state. Huge quantities of chlorine must be added to water to kill bacteria. Almost all cites today increase the toxicity of their water by adding fluoride. Unless you can obtain pure water from a spring or well, your best bet is to purify your own drinking water with a stainless steel water distiller. See "How to avoid drinking doctored water" in Chapter VIII.

Numerous studies made around the world in recent years indicate that people who drink hard water containing calcium have lower fat and cholesterol levels and stand as much as 50 percent less risk of contracting heart disease. Scientists believe that calcium combines with cholesterol and fat molecules, causing them to be eliminated instead of absorbed. For this reason, many people who eat conventional foods are taking 800 mbs. of supplementary calcium daily. Hygienists, of course, consider supplementary calcium unnecessary. For fresh fruits, vegetables, nuts, and seeds are rich in calcium which the body absorbs more readily than in supplement form.

15. Stay mentally active. Because the human mind ages more slowly than any other organ, it is our greatest resource against aging. Given good circulation, our intelligence increases steadily to age fifty and remains constant until at least age eighty. Mental gymnastics can keep your mind sharp and flexible throughout life. Taking college courses or enrolling in adult education classes is an excellent way to keep the mind honed.

Study challenging new subjects. Read the classics and the great works of philosophy. Take up astronomy and cosmology. Learn about the fascinating worlds of botany and biology. Taken an interest in nature. Study a new language. Use your mind to develop new goals and a sense of purpose and direction. Enjoy low-keyed living but always have a fresh life-goal in mind. Maintaining an active mind keeps you younger longer.

At age eighty we are just as productive mentally as at thirty says Dr. Robert Kastenbaum, professor of psychology at the University of Maine. Dr. Kastenbaum advises middle aged people to:

1. Teach someone something every day.
2. Learn something new every day.
3. Enjoy memories, but don't live in the past.
4. Use memory drills and exercise your memory frequently.
5. Meet new people who can converse on fresh subjects.

Dr. Kastenbaum considers keeping the mind youthful and active as one of the most important age-reversing techniques.

16. Lead a happy married life. A survey of 15,000 persons aged eighty and over in the Soviet Union revealed that, with rare exceptions, only married people attain extreme age. In Abkhasia, Professor Pitzkhelauri found couples who had been married seventy years or even longer, and he concluded that marriage and prolonged sex life have an important influence on longevity. Most American centenarians have also experienced decades of marital satisfaction. Another factor linking married life with longevity is Professor Pitzkhelauri's discovery that women who have borne a number of children frequently outlive childless women or women who have only one or two children.

Research by Masters and Johnson proved that sexual response declines negligably between ages thirty and seventy. A number of gerontologists also consider regular sexual activity important in maintaining health during the later years, particularly in men. If you are not currently living happily with a mate, we suggest studying Chapter XI.

17. Live in a healthful environment. All available evidence indicates that people who live in quiet, safe, relaxed smaller towns outlive big city dwellers by several years. Death rates from emphysema and lung cancer are twice as high in industrial cities as in smaller towns. The clatter and hammer of noise in most big cities, and the constant drone of planes over suburbs, is often so emotionally disturbing that it can curtail life and threaten health. To live long, you should move to a quiet, restful place.

But make sure that any small town or rural location you select really *is* quiet. Snowmobiles, speedboats, and roaring trail bikes shatter the peace of many smaller communities while the din of chain saws and other power-driven equipment disturbs the tranquillity of many a rural scene.

We hardly need emphasize that you should live out of reach of pollution of all types. Most of today's centenarians lived the majority of their lives in the pre-chemical, pre-technological decades when the planet was unpolluted. The dramatic rise in the use of chemicals since World War II has produced an epidemic of chemical-related cancers which will only proliferate in forthcoming decades.

If you are free to live where you like, as when you retire, stay as far away as possible from any source of air and water pollution including industries and commercial agriculture.

You can reduce at least part of the hazard of living in the technological age by locating as far away as possible from nuclear power plants, nuclear waste disposal sites, and Air Force bases. You can obtain a free map of Air Force bases entitled *U.S. Active Major Installations* from the U.S. Department of the Air Force, Washington D.C. 20330. A map entitled *Nuclear Power Reactors in the U.S.*, free for the asking from the U.S. Nuclear Regulatory Commission, Washington D.C. 20555, shows the location of all nuclear power plants, existing or proposed. The commission will also send you on request, a map of nuclear waste disposal sites. At every high level atomic graveyard in American, wildlife has already suffered radioactive contamination. These lethal wastes cannot be prevented from leaking out, and they are so dangerous that they are capable of ending all life on earth.

You should also avoid living anywhere in the line of high frequency radiation emanating from such sources as TV and radio towers, microwave transmitters or radar installations, or in close proximity to high voltage power lines.

For complete peace of mind, we would also suggest living outside any area considered a high risk target in a nuclear war. You can obtain a detailed atlas of all high risk target areas by writing the Department of Defense, Defense Civil Preparedness Agency, Washington D.C. 20301, asking for their publication *High Risk Areas.*

Climate doesn't seem to have any appreciable effect on health or longevity. But altitude may make a difference. Though not clinically proven, Canadian biophysicist Dr. Alan Burton recently discovered that the risk of contracting cancer decreases by as much as 50 percent for people living at elevations of 2,000 feet or higher. Dr. Burton's study included ten broad cancer categories and covered the U.S. and other countries around the globe. Throughout the world, the higher the elevation, the lower the rate of cancer mortality.

It is interesting to note that the long-lived peoples of Abkhasia, Vilcabamba, and Hunza all live in mountainous regions at elevations of 5,000 feet or higher. In the U.S., a comparable elevation coupled with a dry, sunny, zestful climate can be found in most of the Southwestern and Rocky Mountain States.

18. Have a twice annual dental check-up, but avoid X-rays. Most people report a sharp decline in dental cavities after becoming Hygienists. But most of us have fillings, crowns, or bridgework that pre-date our conversion to Natural Hygiene. This dental work may become troublesome if not regularly checked. However, you should never agree to be X-rayed unless absolutely unavoidable.

No record is ever kept of the dosage of diagnostic X-rays. Yet every X-ray exposure kills or genetically damages thousands of cells. The dosage is cumulative and as few as 30 rads of radiation has been known to cause leukemia.

A chest X-ray may expose you to .1 rad, a full mouth X-ray to as many as 2.5 rads of lethal radiation concentrated through the mouth and tongue. In retrospect, it may seem almost frightening to recall the many X-rays you may have had and to estimate the total exposure and damage.

Today patients are often subjected to X-rays merely to protect physicians against malpractice suits; or to prove to insurance companies that certain work has been done. Chest X-rays may also be required to qualify for certain occupations. You would be wise to refuse them all.

Try to choose both a doctor and a dentist who are slender and physically fit and who put prevention ahead of surgery and drugs. It's a good general rule to avoid doctors and dentists who smoke and have bad breath, or who are pudgy and have pot bellies and jowels.

For more about X-rays, look up "Radiation—the silent killer" at the end of Chapter II; also "How to prevent cavities by cleaning your teeth the natural way" at the end of Chapter VIII.

13

Inflation-Proof Retirement

The Hygienic Way

Retirement on a fixed income is a disaster for millions of Americans who live and eat conventionally. Inflation, boredom, and declining health are the major threats facing those of us forced to retire at sixty-five. Soaring property taxes and food and utility bills have so impoverished tens of thousands of retirees that they have had to sell their homes and move into apartments or mobile homes. Each year, hundreds of thousands of older couples find they are no longer physically capable of shovelling snow, maintaining yards, or fixing the roof. Those retirees who do have adequate funds often become bored with having nothing to do.

Many Hygienists are able to solve all of these problems by retiring to the Garden Way of Life. By purchasing an easy-to-maintain home with a workshop and large garden in a small, safe, quiet town with low taxes—preferably in a warm Southern state—they often become so self-sufficient that their lifestyle is largely inflation-proof.

When Ray Roberts, a Chicago insurance adjustor, retired at sixty-five, he and his wife Barbara sold their small two-bedroom city home. With the money, they purchased a comfortable, modern home on five acres on the edge of a small retirement town in the Ozarks. Huge trees and lawns surround their charming three-bedroom home which stands on a hill top with a panoramic view. Brick siding reduces the need for painting the house, and since both walls and attic are heavily insulated, heating requirements are minimal.

For months prior to retirement, Ray and Barbara haunted garage sales, accumulating an array of wood and metal household and garden tools. Ray built a workshop in the garage and is able to make all but the most complicated repairs to appliances, furniture, and other belongings. The workshop has cut their repair bills by at least fifty percent.

On moving in, their first task was to plant forty fruit and nut trees and to begin gathering grass and leaves for compost. By the second year, their vegetable garden was supplying Barbara and Ray with well over half of their food needs for the entire year.

Each winter, Barbara and Ray close off all but two rooms in their home, which they heat with electricity supplemented by a wood burning stove. Eventually, the couple plan to build a solar heating system. Their heating costs are less than half of their neighbors, and in summer they use fans instead of air conditioning.

Except during the worst winter weather, Barbara and

Ray make the most of their local trips on foot or by bicycle. Their unmechanized lifestyle keeps them on the go physically for at least eight hours each day. This exercise, coupled with Hygienic eating, protects them from almost all the diseases that plague older Americans.

Their second career as organic gardeners allows Barbara and Ray to work at a satisfying and healthful occupation for the rest of their lives. Their efforts cut their living costs by at least 66 percent all without actually earning any cash, paying taxes, or losing social security benefits. They also barter surplus produce with neighbors for goods and services they may need.

While millions of other Americans retired on fixed incomes are going broke in condominium apartments, or are getting sick from affluent eating, boredom, and physical inactivity, retired Hygienists like Barbara and Ray are having the time of their lives ane enjoying wonderful health besides.

You don't *have* to buy ten acres or retire on a farm to live the Garden Way and to enjoy inflation-proof retirement. Many Hygienic couples simply buy a home in town with a large garden. One eighty-year-old widow of our acquaintance walks eight miles every day and raises trays and jars of sprouts and salad greens in her mobile home. Thousands of retired couples are "farming" fifty-foot lots. Regardless of where you locate, if you live *as if* you were running a self-sufficient homestead, you can protect yourself from most of the risks of ill health, boredom, and inflation.

As the U.S. increasingly commits itself to a philosophy of perpetual prosperity through deficit Goverment spending, the dollar must continually lose value while costs of housing, food, utilities, and services soar. Meanwhile, people are losing faith in the Government, the medical profession, and the food and drug industries. A huge army of compulsorily retired people, supported by a workforce only 3.2 times as large, is steadily bankrupting the Social Security system. By the year 2,000, one American in seven will be over sixty-five, and there will be only 2.5 persons working for every one retired. Social Security payroll taxes to support the swelling ranks of the retired will soon place an insupportable burden on the workforce.

Increasing numbers of Americans are realizing that the only way to count on health and security during the later years is to depend entirely on themselves. In these uncertain times, the Garden Way of Life offers an ideal solution to the day when cancer becomes the number one killer and a pound of hamburger costs $100.

The widespread yearning for a return to the basic values of the natural lifestyle is not limited to retirees. Couples of every age are giving up the urban life to go back to the land. Most Hygienists view the transformation not as retiring *from* a job but as retiring *to* an exciting new career in the world's oldest and most healthful occupation.

Many civic and industrial organizations today allow employees to retire as early as age fifty-five. No one denies the healthful value of work. Yet if your job involves tensions and pressures, the daily stress of commuting, and the risks of working in a polluted environment, you may be better off retiring early to the Garden Way of Life. The younger you are, the easier you'll find it to change to a new occupation. You'll have more time for your fruit trees to grow. And many experts believe that the sooner you take your retirement income, and the sooner you invest your nest egg in a house and land, the more it will buy.

Through observing the retirement scene since 1950, we have witnessed reams of advice in books and magazines on how to retire successfully. Keep active. Take up hobbies. Exercise moderately every day. Sell your stocks and invest in bonds. All these may have some validity. But all overlook the fact that in any successful retirement program, the achievement and maintenance of good health should be given *absolute priority*. With good health achieved through completely natural methods, without dependence on drugs or medical treatment, anyone of any age can successfully combat such problems as boredom and inflation. Health is our most prized possession and its preservation *must* be the cornerstone of any successful retirement plan. For the Garden Way is out of reach of those who are not already fit and healthy when they retire.

If you already own a home with a sizable garden in a quiet, safe, and unpolluted area, you might well consider staying where you are. But most city dwellers will move at retirement. Areas like North and Central Florida, the Gulf Coast, Southeast Texas, and the Ozarks are filled with small, safe towns where taxes are reasonable, the weather mild, and rainfall in excess of forty inches annually. Neither Florida nor Texas currently has a state income tax.

Provided you can rely on irrigation for gardening, you will also find inexpensive small towns dotted all over the Sunbelt States, that arc of popular retirement country that sweeps around the perimeters of the U.S. from Washington to Oregon, California, Arizona, Texas, Utah, and Colorado and on into the Gulf States, Florida, and the South. Away from the big unmanageable cities, scores of small peaceful towns dot the Sunbelt—towns where a woman can walk safely on the streets at two a.m., and you can leave your car unlocked with the keys in the ignition.

The ideal town for Hygienic living has a population of 2,500 to 50,000 with a minimum of two competing supermarkets, each with a well stocked produce counter. Avoid any ambitious town that is exhibiting fast growth. Any tranquillity that remains will soon be destroyed by expansion and endless tax problems, and by eventual congestion, pollution, and crime.

Because of the preponderence of students on bicycles, bicycle riding is usually safe in college towns. Approximately one college in five today offers retirees a chance to audit courses on a noncredit, space-available basis either free or at nominal cost. Larger campuses provide a year-round program of sports, lectures, concerts, and cultural fare at nominal admissions. Natural foods are widely available in college towns and geared to student budgets. Except for homes, land, and property taxes, living costs in college towns tend to be lower.

Independence From Your Own Backyard.

Through intensive cultivation you can grow a satisfying amount and variety of fruits and vegetables on a 25 by 50 foot plot. But for greater variety, and to keep you fully occupied, your lot should be larger, 100 by 400 feet or more if available. You will need space for several compost heaps, and you should plant the perimeter with a variety of fruit and nut trees.

Decide which vegetables suit you most, and plant several long rows of each. A different variety of lettuce can be planted every two weeks from spring through fall. A fresh row of Chinese Cabbage can be sown every three to four weeks. Cold frames and a thick mulch of protective straw can extend growing seasons by weeks. In places like Northern Vermont, Hygienists have produced fresh vegetables for eight months of the year.

Our own list of vegetables includes several rows each of kohlrabi, carrots, beets, Brussell sprouts, broccolli, cauliflower, and several varieties of cabbage. Other parts of the garden are set aside for peas and beans, rhubarb, strawberries, raspberries, blueberries, and currants. We grow three types of grapes, and we have young apple, pear, plum, peach, and cherry trees, some already bearing after only a few years. Each fall, we reap huge crops of delicious honeydew and canteloupe melons, squash of all types, potatoes, turnips, rutabagas, onions, and cucumbers. Our small 100 by 40 foot vegetable plot more than supplies our needs.

Since canning is anathema to Hygienists, we preserve fruits and vegetables through winter in a cool, underground root cellar. Even below ground, some vegetables must be packed in sawdust. Other vines and vegetables continue to grow while underground. About ten per cent of our produce rots, but the root cellar does preserve the remainder. Meanwhile the root cellar, with three feet of solid earth on top, doubles as a fallout shelter in case of nuclear attack or an accident at a nuclear power plant.

For inflation-proof retirement, try to "lockpin" as many costs as possible at today's prices. Of course, taxes, insurance premiums, and utility costs will continue to climb. But most people's Social Security benefits, which have have historically risen in step with inflation, should take care of these expenses. A fixed-interest mortgage secures your housing costs at today's prices and can be paid off with ever-cheaper dollars. Whatever other items and equipment you will need during retirement should be purchased as early as possible, preferably second-hand.

With your own tools and some handyman's skill, you can easily tackle a repair job such as re-roofing your home. You can also build a solar heating system, a greenhouse, cold frames, or an extra room on your house. You can repair your own bicylces and do at least some of the routine body and upholstery maintenance on your car. Oil changes can be easily done at home. With an inexpensive multi-range tester, you can tackle most electrical repairs to your car and home.

Naturally, you can't drop out of the economy entirely. You will need occasional clothes, some foods, and perhaps dental care. You may spend money on entertainment and travel. But most Hygienic homesteaders report that once their garden and fruit trees are established, their monthly budget runs about one third that of retired neighbors who live and eat conventionally.

Moreover, Hygienists enjoy a far superior level of health. But these benefits are available only to people who closely follow the Hygienic lifestyle and who appreciate the simple pleasures of uncomplicated living in harmony with Nature.

A few pointers: modern, well insulated homes are usually far more comfortable and easier to maintain than older homes. The best homes were built between 1950 and 1966. In warm, humid states such as Florida, opt only for a home with masonry walls, a concrete slab foundation, and a ceramic tile roof. The ideal maintenance-free house should also have terrazzo floors, awning windows, and wide eaves with very ample roof ventilation. If the Gulf States, termites and dry or wet rot are a constant threat to roofs.

In dry, cool states like Colorado or Northern New Mexico, all-wood construction (or adobe) is best. In four-seasonal climates, make *sure* your walls are insulated. Demand proof, don't take the seller's word for it. Attic insulation is easily added but insulating walls can be expensive. Homes are generally priced 10-20 percent below the national average in areas like North and Central Florida, the Gulf Coast, the Ozarks, Texas, and Southern Arizona.

Plan to heat only the living room, kitchen, and bathroom. These areas should be thoroughly insulated with storm windows and weather-stripped doors. Try to have as many alternative types of heating as possible. Our home can be heated by natural gas, portable electric heaters, or by a wood-burning cast iron stove, and eventually we plan to add solar heat. In Northern Colorado, our bedrooms are unheated. In all but sub-zero weather, we find that two wool blankets and two comforters keep us snugly warm in bed.

Refrigerated air conditioning is more expensive to install, maintain and operate than the average heating system. In the early 1950s, most retirees were quite content with fans. Then came the great low cost energy splurge when central air conditioning was taken for granted. Today people feel apologetic about inviting guests into a home in Florida or Southern Arizona that is not air conditioned. Yet air conditioning is often installed as much for prestige as for comfort. The fact is that anywhere in the humid South, any fit person can keep comfortably cool by staying out of the midday sun and by utilizing

238

breezes and fans. In the drier Southwest, less costly evaporative cooling can keep you adequately cool. Invariably, people who complain of heat and consider air conditioning essential are those who take no exercise, eat a high fat-high, cholesterol diet, are overweight, constrict their blood vessels by smoking cigarettes, and have an advanced state of atherosclerosis.

To obtain the maximum amount of exercise, many Hygienists garden entirely without the aid of power-driven tools or equipment. All cultivation, spading, forking, sawing, grass cutting, compost-mixing, and other tasks is performed entirely by muscle power. For the utmost stretching benefit, we do most of our bending from the hips, with our knees kept straight.

Most heavy garden work is done in spring and fall. For additional exercise at other times, Hygienists jog, walk, swim, paddle a canoe, or ride a bicycle. For swimming, try to locate near an unpolluted lake, river, spring, or the ocean. The heavily chlorinated water in most swimming pools presents a definite cancer risk. It is almost impossible to swim for any distance without swallowing some.

Hard-packed beaches are fine for jogging, especially at low tide. But many American beaches are spongy and soft. We've found good beaches for walking and running in Northeast Florida, the Florida Gulf Coast, and on the Pacific Coast north of Bandon, Oregon.

Florida and the Ozarks offer unlimited opportunities for stillwater canoeing. Opportunities for serious bicycling are good in much of Texas, especially in the hill country west of San Antonio. Other good bicycling locales exist around DeLand and Homestead in Florida; in the Bisbee area of Arizona; in California' San Diego County; in much of New England (except Maine); and in the Front Range of the Colorado Rockies. Rural Ohio, Pennsylvania, and parts of other Midwestern states have quiet backroads for bicycle riding. Elsewhere, roads are often narrow and dangerous. Cross-country skiing is best in New Hampshire, Vermont, Upstate New York, the Colorado Rockies, and the California Sierras. Hiking is best in the Sierras, Cascades, Colorado Rockies, New Hampshire, and in National Forests over the length of the Appalachians.

You'll use less energy if your car is a manual-shift compact or sub-compact station wagon. American makes are usually cheaper to maintain. By retiring to a perennially warm area, you can make additional savings on snow tires and anti-freeze. Wherever you locate, consider the ever increasing cost if you must drive long distances to stores and services.

In much of Florida, water can be found a few feet below the surface. Even homeowners who have city water find it cheaper to use well water for sprinkling. Elsewhere, wells are often more expensive to dig or deepen. Check carefully on the drought record of local wells before planning to rely on well water during retirement. If your well water is derived from a local drainage basin that is free from industrial and commercial pollution, chances are good that the water itself is pure and free from contaminants. Pure well water can save you the cost and trouble of producing distilled water.

It isn't necessary to be isolated to live the Garden Way. You can own a home with a large lot on the edge of a small town and still have street lights and be within walking distance of stores. If you prefer, you can live the Garden Way by joining a Hygienic commune. At Orange Grove Health Ranch, located on a 180-acre citrus grove near Arcadia in South Central Florida, retired Hygienists live in their own mobile homes or in apartments, and garden communally. Though everyone makes a monthly financial contribution, costs are about as low as it is possible to find. Expenses can be further reduced through cooperative work on construction and other tasks. You can write for information to Orange Grove Health Ranch, Box 316, Route 4, Arcadia FL 33821.

From birth through childhood to adulthood and retirement, most human problems stem from the way man ignores the biological needs of his body and lives by a system that gradually ruins his health. Through bucking the system and living as Nature intended us to, Hygienists, students of hatha yoga, Seventy Day Adventists, and people who follow similar holistic health care systems manage to avoid most of the problems that plague the rest of mankind. At no stage in life does Hygienic living pay off more handsomely than after age sixty-five. When most other people are entering their declining years, the average Hygienist is embarking on an exciting new career which will help him outlive his peers by twelve to twenty or more healthful, happy years.

Appendix

Hygienic Educational and Fasting Institutions
Dr. J. M. Brosius
Bay N' Gulf Hygienic Home
18207-09 Gulf Blvd.
Redington Shores FL 33708

Dr. William L. Esser
Esser's Hygienic Rest Ranch
PO Box 161
Lake Worth FL 33460

R. J. Cheatham N.D.
Shangri-La Health Resort
Bonita Springs FL 33923

Dr. Robert Gross
Pawling Health Manor
PO Box 401
Hyde Park NY 12538

Dr. R. J. Scott
Natural Health Institute
Box 8919
Strongsville OH 44136

Dr. Virginia Vetrano
Dr. Shelton's Health School
PO Box 1277
San Antonio TX 78295

David Stry
Villa Vegetariana
PO Box 1228
Cuernavaca, Mexico

Hygienic Practitioners
Dr. Stanley Bass
3119 Coney Island Ave.
Brooklyn NY 11235

Dr. Gerald Benesh
1450 W. Mission Road
San Marcos CA 92069

Dr. Ralph Cinque
Box 703
Campo CA 92006

Hygienic Retirement Community
Orange Grove Health Ranch
Box 316, Route 4
Arcadia FL 33821

Holistic Natural Health Resorts
Dr. Acer's Vita-Dell Spa
13495 Palm Drive
Desert Hot Springs CA 92240

The Moor's Health Spa
12637 Reposo Way
Desert Hot Springs CA 92240

Meadowlark
26126 Fairview Ave.
Hemet CA 92343

Natural Hygiene and Associated Organizations
American Natural Hygiene Society
1920 Irving Park Road
Chicago IL 60613

American Vegan Society
PO Box H
Malaga NJ 08328

North American Vegetarian Society
501 Old Harding Highway
Malaga NJ 08328

Natural Health Organizations
Association for Holistc Health
PO Box 23231
San Diego CA 92123

International Academy of Biological Medicine Inc.
PO Box 31313
Phoenix AZ 85046

Longevity Research Institute
1211 East Cabrillo Blvd.
Santa Barbara CA 93103

La Leche League International
9616 Minneapolis Ave.
Franklin Park IL 60131

Holistic Health and Nutrition Institute
150 Shoreline Highway 31
Mill Valley CA 94941

Bibliography

A.M.A. Committee on Aging. *Retirement: a Medical Philosophy and Approach.* American Medical Association, 1973.

Benet, Sula. *How to Live to be 100.* New York: Dial Press, 1976.

Benson, Herbert, M.D. *The Relaxation Response.* New York: Avon Books, 1976.

Brodeur, Paul, "Microwaves," *The New Yorker,* 13 and 20 December, 1967, p. 000.

Burman, Edgar, M.D. *The Solid Gold Stethoscope.* New York: Macmillan, 1976.

Burton, Alan C. "Cancer and Altitude." *European Journal of Cancer* 11 (1975): 365-371.

Cooper, Kenneth H. *New Aerobics* New York: M. Evans, 1970.

Cooper, Kenneth H, and Cooper, Mildred. *Aerobics for Women.* New York: M. Evans, 1972.

Comfort, Alex. *A Good Age.* New York: Crown, 1976.

Cott, Alan, M.D. *Fasting: the Ultimate Diet.* New York: Bantam, 1975.

Davies, David, M.D. *Centenarians of the Andes.* San Francisco: Anchor Press, 1975.

Denenberg, Herbert S. *A Shopper's Guide to Surgery.* Insurance Department, Commonwealth of Pennsylvania, 1971.

Flatto, Edwin N.D. *Revitalize Your Body With Nature's Secrets.* New York: Arco, 1973.

Ford, Norman D. *Where To Retire On A Small Income.* Greenlawn, New York: Harian, 1977.

Frank, Benjamin S., M.D. *The No-Aging Diet.* New York: Dial Press, 1976.

Fry T.C. *Program for Dynamic Health.* Natural Hygiene Press, 1974.

Galton, Lawrence. *The Silent Disease: Hypertension.* New York: New American Library, 1973.

Graedon, Joe. *The People's Pharmacy.* New York: St. Martin's Press, 1976.

Hrachovec, Josef P., M.D. *Keeping Young and Living Longer.* Los Angeles: Sherbourne Press, 1972.

Illich, Ivan. *Medical Nemesis: The Expropriation of Health.* New York: Pantheon Press, 1976.

Knight, Granville F., M.D. "Role of Nutrition in the Whole Man." *Journal of Holistic Health;* (1975): 106-115

Krist, Donald A., M.D., and Engel, Bernard T., Ph.D. "Learned Control of Blood Pressure in Patients with High Blood Pressure." *Circulation* 51 (1975): 370-378.

La Leche League. *The Womanly Art of Breast Feeding.* La Leche League International Inc.

Laws, Priscilla W. *Medical and Dental X-Rays: A Consumer's Guide to Avoiding Unnecessary Radiation.* Public Citizen Health Research Group, 1974.

Lappé, Frances Moore. *Diet for a Small Planet.* Cambridge, Mass.: Ballantine, 1975.

Lew, Edward A. "High Blood Pressure, Other Risk Factors and Longevity: the Insurance Viewpoint." *American Journal of Medicine,* 55 (1973).

Mae, Eydie. *How I Conquered Cancer Naturally.* Irvine, Calif.: Harvest House Publishers, 1975.

Nader Report. *Turning Garbage into Money.* Health Research Group, 1975.

Nolan, William A. M.D. *Surgeon Under the Knife.* New York: Coward, McCann and Geoghegan Inc., 1976.

"Nutrition—Applied Personally." International College of Applied Nutrition, 1975.

Oden, Rev. Clifford. *Thank God I have Cancer.* New Rochelle, N.Y.: Arlington House, 1976.

Phillips, Roland L. "Role of Lifestyle and Dietary Habits in Risk of Cancer among Seventh Day Adventists." *Summary of* the Conference on Nutrition in the Cause of Cancer 35 (1976): 3513-21, 3541-43.

Pritikin, Nathan; Jon, Leonard; and Hofer, Jack. Live Longer Now. New York: Grosset and Dunlap, 1974.

Reuben, David M.D. The Save Your Life Diet. New York: Random House, 1975.

Ross, Walter S. You Can Quit Smoking in Fourteen Days. Pleasantville, N.Y.: Readers Digest Press, 1974.

Shelton, Herbert M. Numerous references from Dr. Shelton's Hygienic Review, 1966-76.

Shelton, Herbert M. Food Combining Made Easy. Natural Hygiene Press, 1951.

Whelton, Herbert M. Fasting Can Save Your Life. Natural Hygiene Press, 1964.

Spark, Richard M.D. "The Case Against Regular Physicals." New York Times Magazine, July 25, 1976 p. 10.

Storm, Edward L. Prescription Drugs and Their Side Effects. New York: Grosset and Dunlap Inc., 1976.

Tobe, John H. How to Prevent and Gain Remission from Cancer. Provoker Press, 1975.

Tobe, John H. Security from Five Acres. Provoker Press, 1971.

Transcendental Meditation Publication. "Fundamentals of Progress—Scientific Research on the T.M. Program." Maharishi Mahesh University, 1975.

Trop, Jack Dunn. You Don't Have to be Sick. Natural Hygiene Press. 1961.

Whole Health Bulletin, various issues Shelton CT.

INDEX

251